Getting into

Medical School

2025 Entry

Adam Cross and Emily Lucas

29th edition

trotman t

Getting into Medical School 2025 Entry

This 29th edition published in 2024 by Trotman Education, an imprint of Trotman Indigo Publishing Ltd, 21d Charles Street, Bath BA1 1HX

Authors: Adam Cross and Emily Lucas
24th–28th edns: Adam Cross and Emily Lucas
18th–23rd edns: James Barton and Simon Horner
16th–17th edns: Simon Horner
15th edn: Simon Horner and Steven Piumatti

British Library Cataloguing in Publication Data
A catalogue record for this book is available from the British Library

ISBN 978 1 911724 04 9

Printed and bound by 4Edge Ltd, Hockley, Essex

All details in this book were correct at the time of going to press. To keep up to date with all the latest news and updates and to access the online resources that accompany this book, use this QR code or visit **trotman.co.uk/pages/getting-into-online-resources**.

Contents

About the authors

Adam Cross is Vice Principal at MPW Birmingham and has many years' expertise in helping students gain entry onto competitive undergraduate courses, such as dentistry and medicine. He is also the current co-author of Trotman's *Getting into Dental School* guide. In addition to his careers guidance expertise, Adam also helps students with pre-admissions tests such as the University Clinical Aptitude Test (UCAT). Adam is a highly regarded teacher of biology and has 20 years' experience of delivering GCSE and A level courses.

Emily Lucas read medical science at the University of Birmingham before obtaining a master's degree in genomic medicine from Queen Mary, University of London. She currently holds the position of University Support Officer at MPW, and helps students with their university applications, as well as supporting students with pre-admissions tests such as the University Clinical Aptitude Test (UCAT). As well as teaching, Emily is currently undertaking a PhD in neuroscience at the University of Southampton. Emily also teaches biology, and is the current author of Trotman's *Getting into Veterinary School* guide, and co-author of the *Getting into Dental School* guide.

Acknowledgements

We would like to thank MPW and Trotman Education for giving us the opportunity to produce this edition of *Getting into Medical School*. Many thanks are due to all those who have written previous editions.

We would like to thank all of the individuals who have contributed to the book, especially Dr Simon Bramhall, Camrun Shah, Dr Jaideep Dhillon, Usmaan Khan, Anushka Shah, Dr Shreena Thakaria, Lucy Holland, Shifa Puri, Katy Glenn and Faizaah Chishty for their insights into applying to, studying and working in the field of medicine. In addition, we would like to thank Ibrahim Abedin, Layla Ahmed, Zahra Al-Ani and Katy Glenn for allowing us to reproduce their personal statements here as successful examples. We are extremely grateful that these individuals were willing to take time out of their busy schedules to contribute.

We would also like to thank those at UCAS, the British Medical Association and university admissions departments who have supported us by answering our questions regarding statistics and general advice.

Adam Cross and Emily Lucas
December 2023

About this book

This book is divided into 12 main chapters, which aim to cover three major obstacles that would-be doctors may face:

- getting an interview at medical school
- getting a conditional offer
- getting the right A level grades (or equivalent).

The 12 chapters discuss the following:

1. the study of medicine
2. getting work experience
3. deciding where to apply
4. the UCAS application
5. personal statements
6. the interview process
7. current issues that may come up at interview
8. results day
9. non-standard applications
10. fees and funding
11. career opportunities
12. further information.

Chapter 1 gives information on the actual study of medicine, different teaching styles and postgraduate study, as well as possible specialisations and post-degree course options.

Chapter 2 deals with the significance of undertaking work experience and voluntary work, how to make the most of your placements and how to secure them.

Chapter 3 looks at the different aspects that you should consider when choosing a medical school.

Chapter 4 provides information on the more technical aspects of the UCAS application, with key pointers on how to use UCAS Hub and how to prepare for relevant entrance exams such as the UCAT and BMAT.

Chapter 5 gives an insight into how to write an outstanding personal statement, including how to deliver your points effectively and make your application stand out.

Chapter 6 provides advice on what to expect at the interview stage, current topics, issues you may be questioned about and how to come across as a prospective doctor.

Chapter 7 presents some key information on contemporary and topical medical issues, such as the structure of the NHS, diseases that are appearing in the media, and legal issues that have made the headlines in recent years. Knowing about medical issues is a must, particularly if you are called in for an interview.

Chapter 8 looks at the options that you have at your disposal on results day and describes the steps that you need to take if you are holding an offer or if you have been unsuccessful and have not been given an offer.

Chapter 9 is aimed primarily at overseas students and any other 'non-standard' applicants – mature students, graduates, students who have studied arts A levels and retake students (most medical schools consider non-standard applicants). The chapter also includes some advice for those who want to study medicine outside the UK, say, for example, in the US.

Chapter 10 gives some useful information regarding fees and funding for medical students, as well as bursaries and scholarships that are available, while **Chapter 11** looks at career options in medicine.

Finally, in **Chapter 12**, further information is given in terms of courses and further reading. A number of other excellent books are available on the subject of getting into medical school. The contact details of the various medical groups and universities can also be found here. After Chapter 12 a **Glossary** can be found of many of the terms used throughout the book.

The book also contains numerous case studies and examples of material that will reflect to some extent the theme being discussed at that point. We hope that you find these real-life examples illuminating.

Finally, the views expressed in this book, though informed by conversations with staff at medical schools and elsewhere, are our own, unless specifically attributed to a contributor in the text.

If you have any comments or questions arising from this book, the staff of MPW would be very happy to answer them. You can contact us at the address given below. Good luck with your application to medical school!

Adam Cross and Emily Lucas

MPW (Birmingham)
16–18 Greenfield Crescent
Edgbaston
Birmingham B15 3AU
Tel: 0121 454 9637

Introduction

It is unusual for a day to pass without hearing about the NHS. In recent years, it has been the media's soft toy, often vilified, rarely championed and yet the reality is, the system is simply a victim of its own success. Its chronic underfunding was brought to light by the recent coronavirus pandemic, but that event also unified the country in its appreciation for the outstanding work conducted by its frontline staff. Over the past 50 years, the NHS has made enormous strides, and there is more than one convincing reason to confidently argue that it is better now than ever. It has become better at saving people's lives. This is enormously positive, and yet it means its failures become more transparent, as public expectation in the healthcare sector is now at a level whereby people expect to be saved.

This is where you come in, as aspiring doctors, for which there will always be demand. This book is designed to provide you with much of the information required to formulate a successful application to medical school.

A realistic chance

Typically, there are a fixed number of medical school places available each year and so not all candidates can be successful. Many applicants who are rejected are extremely strong candidates, with high grades at GCSE under their belts and personal qualities that would make them excellent doctors. However, many promising applicants do not put themselves in a position whereby they can be given proper consideration, simply because they do not prepare well enough.

Ideally, your preparation should begin at least two years before you submit your application, but if you have come to the decision to apply to study medicine more recently, or if you were unaware of what steps you need to take in order to prepare a strong application, it isn't too late. Even over a relatively short period of time (a few months), you can put together a convincing application.

In 2023, UCAS reported there were 26,820 applicants to study medicine that year. Of these students, 21,810 were new applicants, whereas 5,010 had applied in previous years. Each applicant was battling for one of approximately 7,100 places available at UK medical schools. Because of the sheer number of applicants, already competitive medicine places have become even tougher to obtain as the number of available places has remained consistent.

In October 2023, the Government announced its plans to expand medical school places for 2024 entry, subject to consultation as part of the NHS Long Term Workforce Plan. The 205 places are to be split between Three Counties (Worcester), Brunel and Chester medical schools – which are new and, at the time of writing, without any publicly funded medical places – and the University of Central Lancashire and Edge Hill medical schools. The latter two schools being chosen due to their location in the north-west of England, where additional doctors are most needed.

The grades you need

Table 8 (see pages 214–217) shows that, with a few exceptions, the A level grades you need for medicine are AAA, though there are some A* offers around now. A number of medical schools, including Cambridge, Keele, King's College London, Queen Mary University of London, Oxford, Queen's University Belfast and University College London are asking for an A* grade in their entry offers going forwards. Other universities, such as Plymouth, also state that an A* grade *may* be stipulated as part of their offer. For students who are retaking their A levels, A* grades are often included in offers, such as the University of East Anglia who outline this condition as part of their resit policy.

As a general guide, candidates with qualifications other than A levels are likely to need the following:

- Scottish: AAAAB in Highers or AA in Advanced Highers to include AAAAB in Highers (some universities only consider Advanced Highers)
- International Baccalaureate: around 34–43 points, including 7, 7, 6–6, 6, 5 at Higher level (with most including chemistry)
- European Baccalaureate: roughly 80% overall, with at least 80% in chemistry and another full option science/mathematical subject.

But there's more to it than grades ...

If getting a place to study medicine were purely a matter of achieving the right grades, medical schools would demand A*AA at A level (or equivalent) and 10 top grades at GCSE, and they would not bother to conduct interviews. However, becoming a successful doctor requires many skills, academic and otherwise, and it is the job of the admissions staff to try to identify who of the thousands of applicants are the most suitable. It would be misleading to say that anyone, with enough effort, could become a doctor, but it is important for candidates who have the potential to succeed to make the best use of their applications.

Non-standard and second-time applications

Not all successful applicants apply during their final year of A levels. Some have retaken their exams, while others have used a gap year to add substance to their UCAS application. Again, it would be wrong to say that anyone who reapplies will automatically get a place, but good candidates should not assume that rejection first time round means the end of their medical career aspirations.

Gaining a place as a retake student or as a second-time applicant is not as easy as it used to be, but candidates who can demonstrate genuine commitment alongside the right personal and academic qualities still have a good chance of success if they go about their applications in the right way. The admissions staff at the medical schools tend to be extremely helpful and, except at the busiest points in the year when they simply do not have the time, they will give advice and encouragement to suitable applicants. With this in mind, it is worth conducting your research in good time and contacting universities well before the October application deadline in order to identify the universities to which your application would be best suited.

Admissions

The medical schools make strenuous efforts to maintain fair selection procedures: UCAS applications are generally seen by more than one selector, interview panels are given strict guidelines about what they can (and cannot) ask, and most make detailed statistics available about the backgrounds of the students they interview. Above all, admissions staff will tell you that they are looking for good 'all-rounders' who can communicate effectively with others, are academically capable and are genuinely enthusiastic about medicine – if you think that this sounds like you, then read on!

Steps to prepare you for a successful medicine application

The process of applying for medicine is challenging, so it is vital you take all of the necessary steps required to ensure an excellent chance of securing a place. Before you apply, thoroughly research the stages of the application process and the demands of the course and career.

1. Establish whether medicine is the right career for you
2. Secure relevant work experience and voluntary placements
3. Determine whether you are up to the academic challenge of getting into medicine and studying it
4. Ensure you have the right qualities to make an excellent doctor
5. Identify which universities you might like to study at
6. Research your chosen universities to ensure that the course they offer is suitable for your own learning needs
7. Ascertain the entry requirements for your chosen universities, including academic attainment and pre-admissions testing
8. Identify what makes an outstanding personal statement
9. Develop your interview skills

Reflections of a doctor

The words below from a qualified practitioner and a first-year medical student express and reflect some of the many challenges and rewards that you may also face in your own journey to become a doctor. As with every journey, the grandest ones start with the first minuscule step.

Case study

Faaizah completed a first degree at the University of East Anglia, before studying Medicine at Nottingham. Faaizah is currently working as a Junior Doctor.

'I think everyone's experience of being a medic is slightly different – for me, it's chaotic, exciting and challenging. I love busy days filled with going to theatre and seeing new, innovative treatments. One day I'm in a robotic list, another day in a laser list; getting to scrub in and assist in these cases really excites me and makes the job what it is!

'I love working with people, and a big part of being a trainee in the hospital is being a team player; having trust in and problem solving with all your Multi-Disciplinary Team colleagues is one of the most rewarding parts of the job. Of course, ultimately, nothing compares to helping patients and seeing that your hard work has made a difference or made a difficult journey just a little bit easier.

'Medicine is challenging, and I'm continually learning. Constant juggling of projects, exams and maintaining some sort of work–life balance is demanding, in both brain power and physical time.

'Prospective medics need to be aware that they will be challenged with time management, imposter syndrome and constant decision fatigue!

'As a junior doctor, every day is different and there are lots of both ups and downs; there are tough situations, but you get to see where your strengths and interests lie, and hopefully it leads to a speciality where you really enjoy what you do. It's a brilliant, rewarding (definitely exhausting) career.

'The teams I have worked with have made the job very rewarding – I have been lucky enough to work with some of the nicest people; the knowledge and advice they have imparted has been invaluable.

'However, there are some challenging aspects of the job. There are lots of days when you end up taking your work home with you – for me, this is usually thoughts about how I've cared for a patient or if I've done my best that day. It's times like these when having a good team around you helps you process your thoughts.

'The (first) peak of the pandemic meant that I remained in my job in elderly care, rather than rotating on to my next placement. Covid-19 hit the elderly patients harder than we were initially expecting. The loss of patients and staff was significant. The difficult conversations I had to have with patients and their families, I do not think I would have experienced outside of this situation. Compassion and empathy had never been more important.

'My biggest tip for aspiring medics is to make sure that you really want a career in medicine. It is not easy and it is not glamorous. There is a lot of work to be done, and at times the system can be frustrating. However, the experiences you will have will be like no other. I cannot see myself doing anything else.'

Case study

Katy is a first-year medical student at the University of Bristol. Katy had initially opted to study English and French at the University of Warwick before deciding that she wanted to pursue a career in medicine.

'I think that medicine is a very special degree. It is so much more than just the study of the body, health and disease – you are also learning how to be a good, compassionate and competent doctor, which encompasses learning skills in consultation, anatomy, biology, ethics, behavioural and social sciences, and lots more! You are committing to a career that involves lifelong learning and gives you the opportunity to specialise in too many areas to count or to get involved in so many other aspects of healthcare, such as research or teaching. As a degree, and a future career it is very people-focused, and it allows you to put your knowledge and skills to use on a daily basis to help people – I think this is the main reason why I chose to study medicine, as I was really attracted to the idea of studying something that I was not only interested in, but that I could also visualise using my knowledge in the future to help individuals.

'Before applying, I worked part time at a GP surgery in an administrative role for a couple of months; carried out a couple of weeks' work experience in two different hospitals local to me, which gave me the opportunity to shadow a range of healthcare professionals; and worked as a domiciliary carer for a month.

'My work experience cemented my desire to study medicine; it showed me some of the benefits and the difficult realities of working in healthcare and as a doctor. Working as a carer in particular was valuable in improving my empathy and my communication skills, and gave me an insight into the day-to-day life of people living with complex health needs and disability; this experience is really beneficial for applying to study medicine as it gave me a lot of exposure to different health needs and how they are managed at home – this gave me a lot to talk about at interview as well!

'I had a slightly unusual journey into medicine. When I originally took my A levels, I studied English Literature, History and French and then went to university to study for a degree in English Literature and French. During the university holidays, I worked part time at a GP surgery, where I discovered that I really wanted to study medicine, and work as a doctor! I left university after my first year, and studied for A levels in Biology and Chemistry in the condensed period of one year, so that I could apply to study medicine. After studying and securing my grades, I had a year out while I was applying to medical school, during which I worked as a carer and then as a healthcare assistant in a hospital – this has been really valuable experience for me, as I have now had a lot of contact with patients, and improved my communication skills and confidence.

'I am particularly enjoying how varied the course is, and how it is so focused on patient-centred care. I am really enjoying learning about Behavioural Social Sciences – where we are learning about things such as health behaviours and the patient–doctor relationship. I am only a few weeks into the course, however and I am sure there will be so many more aspects that I enjoy in the future! However, medicine is an incredibly vast subject, and it can be easy to feel a bit overwhelmed by the huge amount of information that is out there to learn.

'I think it's too early in the course to tell what I'll want to specialise in, but I'm excited to discover different areas of medicine and find what I am particularly interested in, and may want to specialise in, in the future.

'It can be a really daunting experience applying to medical school, and it is easy to let worries about interviews and offers get you down. Remember that you are unique and have something different to offer than other applicants! Do your research, and practise answering interview questions with friends and family, but also remember that more often than not, at interview they want to see that you are enthusiastic and able to have a genuine conversation with someone, and they want to learn more about you, your experience and your values – having set answers and rehearsed responses will not help with that! I would also say to really think about which medical school will be a good fit for you – whether you would learn best from a traditional medicine course, or an integrated course with early patient contact, whether you are excited by the thought of case-based or problem-based learning – each course is unique so it's important to do your research, and this will also help with answering questions at interview as well.'

1 | Studying medicine

This chapter mainly discusses studying medicine as an undergraduate course. For information on postgraduate courses, see the section entitled 'Postgraduate courses' on page 25.

Medical courses are carefully planned by the General Medical Council (GMC) to give students a wide range of academic and practical experience, which will lead to final qualification as a doctor. The main difference between medical schools is the method of teaching. At the end of the five-year course, students will – if they have met the high academic standards demanded – be awarded a Bachelor of Medicine (MB) or Bachelor of Medicine and Surgery (MBBS or MBChB). Degrees in medicine are regarded as professional degrees and, as such, are not honours degrees (also, there are no classes, e.g. 2.i, 2.ii, etc., but simply pass or fail). However, medicine degrees can be awarded with honours for truly exceptional performance, but this is unusual. In such cases '(Hons)' is added to the degree designation.

It is well worth noting that, at this stage, doctors are graduates and have yet to specialise. To become a consultant involves training and developing for years in a chosen specialism.

Teaching styles

The structure of all medical courses is similar, with most institutions offering two years of pre-clinical studies followed by three years of clinical studies. However, schools differ in the ways in which they deliver the material, so it is very important to thoroughly check the course information of each university to which you are thinking of applying.

Medical courses can be classified as either traditional, problem-based learning (PBL), case-based learning (CBL), team-based learning (TBL) or integrated. The table overleaf shows a list of the medical schools in the UK along with the teaching style they practise.

As you will see from the example course descriptions, all medical school courses cover the same essential information but can vary widely in their teaching styles; this is an important point to consider when choosing which course to apply to. Chapter 3 has further guidance on what to consider when choosing your university and course.

Table 1 Teaching styles

Medical school	Teaching style
University of Aberdeen	Integrated
Anglia Ruskin University	Integrated
Aston University	Integrated
Barts and The London School of Medicine and Dentistry (Queen Mary University of London)	PBL
University of Birmingham	Integrated (including CBL)
Brighton and Sussex Medical School	Integrated
University of Bristol	Integrated
Brunel University	TBL
University of Buckingham	Integrated
University of Cambridge	Traditional
Cardiff University	CBL
University of Central Lancashire	Integrated
University of Dundee	Integrated
University of East Anglia	Integrated
University of Edinburgh	Integrated
University of Exeter	Integrated
University of Glasgow	Integrated (including PCL and CBL)
Hull York Medical School	PBL
Imperial College London	Integrated
Keele University	Integrated
Kent and Medway	Integrated
King's College London	Integrated
Lancaster University	PBL
University of Leeds	Integrated
University of Leicester	Integrated
University of Lincoln	Integrated
University of Liverpool	Integrated (including CBL)
University of Manchester	PBL
Newcastle University	Integrated
University of Nottingham	Integrated
University of Oxford	Traditional
University of Plymouth	PBL
Queen's University Belfast	Integrated
University of St Andrews	Integrated
St George's, University of London	Integrated
University of Sheffield	Integrated
University of Southampton	Integrated
University of Sunderland	PBL
University College London	Integrated
Swansea University	Integrated
University of Warwick	Integrated
University of Worcester	PBL

Traditional courses

This is the more long-established, lecture-based style, using didactic methods such as lectures as a means of delivering the information. Generally, they have a structure that consists of two or three years of taught theory, followed by two to three years of clinical training. It has to be said that these courses are a rarity today and are limited to establishments such as Cambridge and Oxford, where there is a definite pre-clinical/clinical divide and the pre-clinical years are taught very rigidly in subjects.

TIP!

Find out more details about these traditional-based learning courses by going to the websites for the following medical schools:

- University of Oxford: www.medsci.ox.ac.uk
- University of Cambridge: www.medschl.cam.ac.uk

Course structure: Cambridge (Traditional)

Cambridge's medicine courses are intellectually stimulating and professionally challenging. They provide rigorous training in the medical sciences, while equipping students with the communication, interpersonal and clinical skills required by today's doctors.

Years 1, 2 & 3

As is typically the case with traditionally taught courses, at Cambridge, students are taught the medical sciences for the first three years, which are referred to as pre-clinical studies.

Pre-clinical studies involve around 20–25 timetabled hours per week, which includes taught lectures, practical classes (such as dissections) and supervisions.

In years 1 and 2, the main academic areas covered include Functional Architecture of the Body, Homeostasis, Molecules in Medical Science, Biology of Disease, Mechanisms of Drug Action, Neurobiology and Human Behaviour and Human Reproduction. These are designed to give you an excellent foundation in medical sciences.

You will also study a clinical strand, including an Introduction to the Scientific Basis of Medicine, Social Context of Health and Illness and Preparing for Patients. While the main focus is academic during this period of the degree, the Preparing for Patients Module eases into the clinical aspects of medicine through patient interaction in a GP surgery in year 1, a hospital setting in year 2 and through visiting community-based health-related agencies in year 3.

The third year of the course allows you to specialise in an alternative subject – a process known as intercalation. Students can choose from a wide variety of subjects, such as pathology, physiology, zoology, psychology and natural sciences, or even a subject that is entirely distinct from medicine, such as anthropology, management studies or philosophy.

Upon successful completion of the first three years, you will be awarded a BA degree in your chosen subject.

Years 4, 5 & 6

The subsequent three years of a Cambridge medicine course involve learning predominantly in clinical settings, such as GP surgeries and outpatient clinics. By this point, you will be thoroughly equipped with medical knowledge, and therefore the clinical component of the course provides a crucial opportunity to develop bedside skills. These clinical sessions are supported by seminars, tutorials and discussion groups.

Clinical studies are based at the Cambridge Biomedical Campus and Cambridge University Hospitals NHS Foundation Trust, as well as a variety of other regional NHS hospitals throughout the East of England and general practices in Cambridge.

The clinical studies aim to enhance your biomedical knowledge while allowing you to hone your practical skills and attitudes required to practise clinical medicine. Each of the three years has its own focus: year 4 – core clinical practice, year 5 – specialist clinical practice, and year 6 – applied clinical practice. Each of these is based around several major themes, including communication skills, patient investigation and practical procedures; therapeutics and patient management; core science, pathology and clinical problems; evaluation and research and professionalism and patient safety.

In addition, you will also have weekly clinical supervisions. These small group sessions with junior doctors are designed to assist with the further development of your clinical skills.

After successful completion of the clinical years, you will be awarded the Bachelor of Medicine and the Bachelor of Surgery degree (MB, BChir) in addition to your BA degree.

Assessment

Assessment is continuous throughout all six years, and progress is reviewed weekly and termly by college supervisors. Formal assessments comprise written and practical examinations, coursework submission and clinical assessments. Only upon successful completion of these tasks can you progress with the course.

Problem-based learning (PBL)

The PBL course, commended by the GMC, was pioneered by medical schools such as Liverpool (which now offers an integrated course) and Manchester and subsequently taken up by a number of other medical schools such as Plymouth and Hull York. The course is taught with a patient-oriented approach. From year 1 onwards, students are heavily involved in clinical scenarios, with the focus on the student to demonstrate self-motivation and proactive, self-directed learning, both independently and as part of a small group. This type of teaching and learning is designed to get away from the previous traditional 'spoon-fed' approach; therefore, those who are used to the spoon feeding of information may take some time to adjust.

It is common now for medical schools to utilise PBL to varying levels. Some will use PBL sessions as a predominant learning tool, supplemented by lectures, whereas others will utilise them around taught content periodically.

A typical PBL session involves dissecting a case study, or 'problem', as part of a small group. Once you have been presented with this information, it is down to your group to decide what you will need to learn to handle the situation before going away and discovering it for yourselves, and then feeding back to your group coordinator. The idea is that you acquire knowledge through research-based problem solving, rather than being taught directly.

Studying at Peninsula Medical School, University of Plymouth

Students benefit from close relationships with several NHS hospital partners, where they practise their clinical and communication skills in the safe setting of Plymouth's Clinical Skills Resource Centre (CSRC). The CSRC features specially designed replicas of hospital wards and emergency rooms, with high specification patient-simulators. You will also learn from real patients from the outset, with clinical placements starting in the first two weeks of year one.

Years 1 & 2

In the first two years, students learn the core scientific foundations of medicine within a clinical context. In the first year, the curriculum is structured around the human life cycle, so in that year, human physical and psychological development from conception to old age are studied. Students will learn from real-life clinical case studies and experience healthcare in a range of community settings, meeting patients and service users, and learning from health and social care professionals.

In the second year, the human life cycle is revisited, this time with an emphasis on disease, pathological processes and the human and social impact of illness and disease. Students undertake a series of placements in a single general practice, enabling them to learn about long-term health issues and see teamwork in action.

The modules covered over these two years include Medical Knowledge, Clinical and Communication Skills, Personal Development and Professionalism and a Student-Selected Component.

Years 3 & 4

In Years 3 and 4, students will learn more about clinical practice and spend more time in a patient-centred learning environment. Completing a series of hospital and general practice-based community placements, students will gain valuable experience in a wide range of clinical settings and see first-hand how the NHS works as a team to deliver patient care.

Year 3 focuses on three Pathways of Care: Acute Care, Ward Care and Integrated Ambulatory Care.

In their fourth year, students will continue working and learning in hospital and general practice settings, further developing their communication, clinical, problem-solving and analytical skills. The three Pathways of Care continue in year four with a focus on Acute Care, Palliative Care, Oncology and Continuing Care.

Year 5

Students will now be in a position to apply the knowledge, skills and confidence they have acquired over the first four years by working 'on the job', as part of a healthcare team in action, based in either Derriford or Torbay hospital. Students become more assured when dealing with clinical situations, and develop an in-depth understanding of the principles of practice in the NHS. Supplementing their independent learning with a portfolio of indicative presentations, students will also have the opportunity to do an elective in a different social or cultural context.

PBL example

The Peninsula Medical School at the University of Plymouth follows an eight-step process, built on the literature and the school's own experience of how students learn in its setting. The eight steps are designed to develop your learning skills to ensure you are prepared for the clinical environment, where you will be faced with many new and unfamiliar situations. In doing so, PBL will help prepare you for life as a foundation doctor. The curriculum follows the life cycle, and PBL cases build in complexity to allow you to integrate and consolidate your understanding of the topics and concepts introduced in other parts of the course. Each PBL case lasts for two weeks and includes three two-hour sessions and follows an unfolding case. In PBL you will draw on your learning from other parts of the course, including small-group and lecture-style components. The final PBL session allows you to consolidate new learning and apply what you have learned to new patient scenarios.

The key learning outcomes for PBL at Peninsula Medical School include the development of transferable learning skills required for lifelong learning and applicable to your life and career as a doctor, including:

- critical thinking
- understanding uncertainty
- working with complexity
- being comfortable with the limits of knowledge
- team working.

A typical example of a case scenario would be:

Mr Ted Bryce is a fifty-eight-year-old man who comes to see you (his GP), because he has been having trouble sleeping for a few months and would like some sleeping tablets.

You ask him some questions to try to find out about his insomnia and you discover: he has four children, two of whom are still at school; he works for a local engineering company, which is threatened with closure, and he feels stressed that he might lose his job and will not be able to feed his family and his house might be repossessed.

You look on the computer at his medical records and discover that he was put on medication to treat high blood pressure two years ago, but that he hasn't requested a repeat prescription for almost a year.

You check his blood pressure and find that it is a bit high.

Figure 1 Process

- Read the scenario and
- Ensure everybody understands the language used

- Brainstorm the issues raised by the case
- Group them according to main themes

- Determine students' prior knowledge and understanding of each of the issues
- Develop a concept map

- Identify gaps in knowledge and understanding
- Develop 'SMART' questions that promote understanding and contextualisation

- Research questions as individuals or in groups during personal study time

- Report findings to the group
- Discuss difficult concepts
- Add new learning to the concept map of the case

- Consider new learning within the context of the case
- Think about how these might apply to similar/different cases e.g. what if...? questions

- Reflect on how the group and individual members performed within the group
- Feed back what went well and what could be improved

To work through this scenario, your group will identify the main issues from the case and group them into themes. You will then consider what you already know (activate prior knowledge), using concept maps (see Figure 2).

Figure 2 Concept maps

1) identify the issues

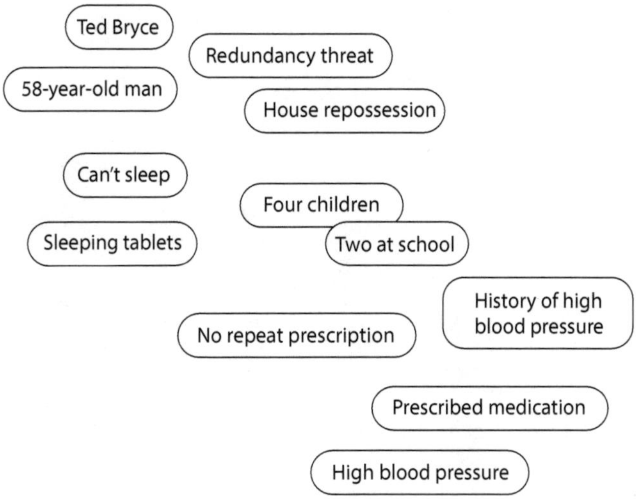

2) Group into themes

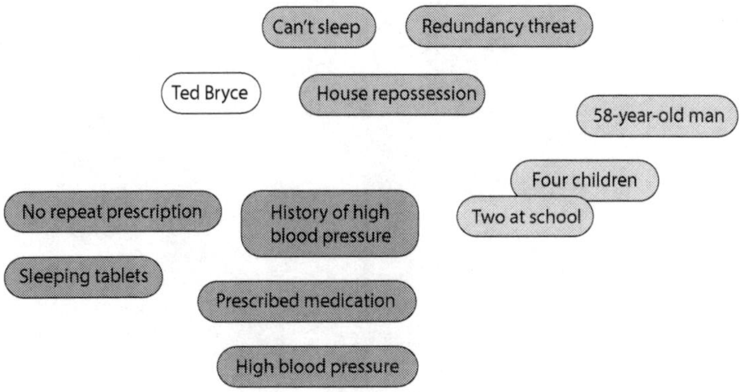

This process will also help you recognise what you don't know and set questions to develop your understanding e.g.

1. Why does narrowing of the arteries cause blood pressure to go up?
2. How do arteries become narrower?
3. How is fluid volume controlled in the body?
4. Why do people become stressed?
5. What can doctors do to help people manage stress?

6. How does stress affect sleep?
7. Why don't people take their medication?
8. How can we manage screening of all the people in the local area with high blood pressure?

Some of the issues raised will be addressed in some of the other learning sessions and some will require you to do some research, or look back at things you have done earlier in the year. The main aim is to get you thinking like a doctor and working out what you would need to know in order to help the patient and the wider population.

3) Activate prior knowledge

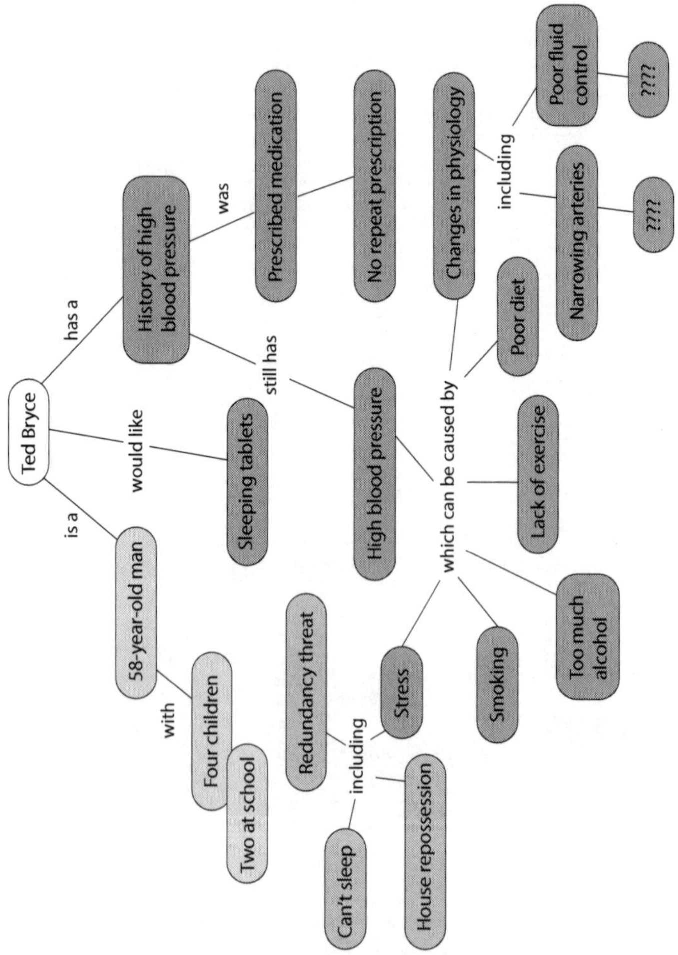

With thanks to Dr Kerry Gilbert, University of Plymouth – Lead for PBL. Reprinted with the kind permission of the Peninsula Medical School, University of Plymouth.

Integrated courses

Integrated courses are those where basic medical sciences are taught concurrently with clinical studies. Thus, this style is a combination of a traditional course and a PBL course and, currently, is the most common type of medical course. Although these courses have patient contact from the start, there is huge variation in the amount of contact from school to school. In Year 1, contact is quite often limited to local community visits, with the amount of patient contact increasing as the years progress. In any case, most students are quite happy with having only limited contact with patients in the first year, as they feel that at this point they do not have a sufficient clinical knowledge base to approach patients on the wards.

With clinical training taking place alongside taught theory, students are able to develop both their knowledge and clinical aptitude side by side. It is an approach that is thoroughly endorsed by the General Medical Council and is therefore adopted by a large number of universities.

Studying at the University of Exeter Medical School (integrated)

Throughout the duration of the medicine programme at the University of Exeter, students will study in a variety of clinical locations across the South West: in hospitals, general practice and the wider health community.

The core curriculum delivers the essential knowledge and skills for your role as a newly qualified doctor while allowing you a degree of freedom in choosing a wide range of Student Selected Special Study Units that amount to approximately one-third of the programme. Exposure to the clinical environment begins in the first week and hands-on community experience increases throughout the degree. The programme integrates medical science and clinical skills so that your academic learning is applied to clinical practice throughout the five years.

The programme is designed around a core curriculum that provides the essential foundation of knowledge required for practising newly qualified doctors. The University of Exeter also offers a range of Student Selected Special Study Units, which allows the student to select preferential modules as part of their training to tailor their learning experience.

In terms of clinical experience, patient contact starts immediately, with a progressive increase in time commitment throughout the programme. Clinical contact takes place alongside taught medical science to allow learning to be applied in real time.

Years 1 & 2

For the first year, students will be based at the St Luke's Campus, Exeter, and will experience university life to the full. Taught modules focus on core biomedical and psychosocial content, which can be applied in the clinical placements that run alongside. There is also committed clinical skills training.

This learning is built upon in the second year with further teaching in core concepts, including biomedical, psychological, sociological and population health. Studying continues to be integrated alongside clinical placements and clinical skills training.

Years 3 & 4

During the third year, patient-centred learning is increased, with more time spent on hospital and community placement rotations, which will be located in either Devon or Cornwall. This period of training is known as Clinical Pathways 1.

Clinical Pathways 2 follows in the fourth year, where further clinical placements in a wider range of settings and specialities are undertaken in order to improve clinical knowledge and skills.

Year 5

In the fifth year, learning is largely clinical placement-based to allow students to develop their own practice in readiness for life as a newly qualified doctor through apprenticeship attachments in various hospitals. This will provide extensive experience of working as part of a healthcare team in a clinical environment in real time, and give rise to ample opportunities to practise interpreting diagnostic tests and implementing patient management plans.

The learning and experiences from years 1–4 should put fifth-year students in a strong position for analysing and evaluating patient conditions, as well as for suggesting clinical management plans. Students will also undertake either a research or clinical-based Elective, either in the UK or abroad. This will provide an opportunity to broaden a student's exposure to medicine.

Case-based learning

This is not the same as problem-based learning, though its ideals are similar. Unlike PBL, which is focused on problem-based scenarios, case-based learning looks at case studies within a clinical environment. It is actually quite a common route for a lot of international medical schools, and has more recently been implemented by a number of UK medical schools such as Cardiff University. In addition, the University of Glasgow and the University of Liverpool have integrated the CBL approach into their curriculum to some extent. It is a popular way of learning, with a US poll among 286 students and 31 faculties displaying an 89% preference for the CBL teaching methods.

The style of teaching will be in small groups and utilises clinical cases to elicit interest in and discussion of a specific part of the course curriculum. Within these sessions, activities will be carried out with a plenary session at the end for students to share their experiences and discuss the application of them in the future.

It is expected this type of learning will become more popular in the UK sooner rather than later, with more universities starting to use this style of teaching.

Case-based learning at the University of Warwick

The University of Warwick uses case-based learning, a learner-centred approach to the study of medicine, at the core of its curriculum. Considered as a process of directed discovery, case-based learning encourages students to identify what it is that they need to learn about medicine, and how they can learn it, when reflecting on a patient case, while also drawing on their prior knowledge and experience.

Case-based learning has been adopted by the University of Warwick as it supports students in integrating their knowledge of medicine across biomedical, social and clinical sciences; providing an opportunity to apply this knowledge in a clinical context, for the development of problem solving and clinical reasoning skills and the development of skills required for practising medicine, including team work, communication, professional skills and those for self-directed learning.

Team-based learning

Brunel University has recently opened a medical school for international students, and delivers its teaching through a method they have termed Team-Based Learning (TBL), which is a variation on PBL and CBL. As the name suggests, TBL encourages teamwork, which is a crucial skill in medicine. It allows for the development of collaboration skills and the ability to take on board and provide constructive feedback for continued development. TBL also involves students receiving learning materials in advance of teaching sessions, so that they can process the information in advance before working through problems in their groups based on the content as a means of enhancing learning retention.

Intercalated degrees

Students who perform well in the examinations at the end of their pre-clinical studies (year 2 or 3) often take up the opportunity to complete an intercalated degree. An intercalated degree gives you the opportunity to incorporate a further degree (BSc or BA) into your medical course. This is normally a one-year project, during which students have the opportunity to investigate a chosen topic in much more depth, producing a final written thesis before rejoining the main course. Usually, a range of degrees are available to choose from, such as those from the traditional sciences, e.g. biochemistry, anatomy, physiology, or in topics as different as medical law, ethics, journalism or history of medicine.

The University of Manchester, for example, offers intercalated degrees to its third- and fourth-year MBChB students as an opportunity to acquire new skills in a different kind of study. Intercalating students can choose to study from a range of undergraduate courses, including Anatomical Sciences, Biochemistry, Biomedical Sciences, Cell Biology, Developmental Biology, Genetics, Global Health, Immunology, Medical Biochemistry, Neuroscience, Pharmacology and Physiology, and Medical Physiology.

One of the most popular choices for intercalation is biomedical or clinical science. As these are research-based degrees, they provide the opportunity for medical students to enhance their scientific knowledge of an area of interest, such as neuroscience or reproductive biology, as content is often covered at a deeper level than on a medicine degree. It also gives medical students an opportunity to participate in medical research and, in some cases, may even provide a chance to secure publications.

Why intercalate?

- It gives you the chance to study a particular subject in depth.
- It gives you the chance to be involved in research or lab work, particularly if you are interested in research later on.
- It gives you an advantage over other candidates if you later decide to specialise; for example, intercalating in anatomy would be useful if you wish to pursue a career in surgery.

Why not intercalate?

If you're not interested in studying beyond a medical degree and practising as a doctor, then you might decline the opportunity to intercalate. Intercalating will increase the number of years that you end up studying, and there is an additional cost associated with this too.

TIP!

Websites with further information about intercalated degrees:

- www.intercalate.co.uk
- www.qmul.ac.uk/fmd/study/undergraduate/courses/intercalated (Barts and The London School of Medicine and Dentistry)
- www.kcl.ac.uk/study/subject-areas/intercalated/intercalated-bsc-courses (King's College London)
- www.bma.org.uk/advice-and-support/studying-medicine/becoming-a-doctor/intercalated-degrees (British Medical Association)
- www.healthcareers.nhs.uk/explore-roles/doctors/medical-school/intercalated-medical-degrees (NHS Health Careers)
- www.liverpool.ac.uk/medicine/study-with-us/intercalation (University of Liverpool School of Medicine)

Taking an elective

Towards the end of the course there is often the opportunity to take an elective study period, usually for two months, when students are expected to undertake a short project but are free to travel to any hospital or clinic in the world that is approved by their university. This gives you the opportunity to practise medicine anywhere in the world during your clinical years. For example, electives range from running clinics in developing countries to accompanying flying doctors in Australia. Students see this as an opportunity to do some travelling and visit exotic locations far from home before they qualify. You can also opt to do an elective at home. If you want to know more about this, go to www.worktheworld.co.uk.

Postgraduate courses

There is a huge variety of opportunities and courses for further postgraduate education and training in medicine. This reflects the array of possible areas for specialisation. Medical schools and hospitals run a wide range of postgraduate programmes, which include further clinical and non-clinical training and research degree programmes. Such courses include masters and PhD programmes in fields ranging from cancer immunology to health psychology to regenerative medicine, so it is possible to undertake postgraduate study in highly specialised areas.

Advice and guidance are available from the Royal College of Physicians (RCP) (www.rcplondon.ac.uk) and the individual universities. As before, you will need to check the prospectuses of individual universities for the most up-to-date information.

Examples of postgraduate courses

The following are postgraduate degrees in the field of medicine:

- Respiratory Medicine, MSc, University of Birmingham
- Advanced Clinical Practice (Acute Medicine), MSc, University of Bolton
- Precision Medicine, MSc, University of Glasgow
- Internal Medicine, MSc, University of Edinburgh
- Reproductive Medicine (Science and Ethics), MSc, University of Kent
- Tropical Paediatrics, MSc, Liverpool School of Tropical Medicine
- Regenerative Medicine and Stem Cells, MRes, Newcastle University
- Emergency and Resuscitation Medicine, MSc, Queen Mary University of London
- Cancer Medicine, MSc, Queen's University Belfast
- Nutritional Medicine, MSc, University of Surrey
- Genomic Medicine, MSc, Swansea University
- Genetics and Multiomics in Medicine, MA, UCL
- Translational Cardiovascular Medicine, MSc/PgCert/PgDip, University of Bristol
- Health, Medicine and Society, MPhil, University of Cambridge
- Extreme Medicine, MSc/PgCert/PgDip, University of Exeter
- Law, Medicine and Healthcare, LLM, University of Liverpool
- Genomics and Experimental Medicine, PhD, University of Edinburgh
- Tropical Health and Infectious Disease Research, PhD, Liverpool School of Tropical Medicine
- Medicine and Surgery, PhD, Newcastle University

Case study

Dr Shreena Thakaria is a junior doctor. After completing her undergraduate degree in Medical Science at the University of Birmingham, she studied postgraduate Medicine at the University of Limerick in Ireland.

'I am currently doing my foundation years in East Anglia. My F1 was in Ipswich hospital and my F2 is currently in Norwich. I have done rotations in Care of the Elderly, General Surgery and Orthogeriatrics. I am currently on Trauma and Orthopaedics, and am due to carry out rotations in General Practice and Ear, Nose and Throat.

'The Trauma and Orthopaedics department is very busy. It is definitely multidisciplinary, as I work alongside the consultants, nurse practitioners, registrars, core surgical trainees, nurses, Health Care Assistants, OPM team (geriatricians), physiotherapists and pharmacists. I find my role is "continuity of care" – as the Senior House Officer, I'm the person who spends the most amount of time on the wards and in the Emergency Department clerking the patients and looking after them once they're admitted; I then fill in the other members of the team about the patient's baseline mobility pre-fall, their regular medications and any co-morbidities that might interfere with surgery. I also update the next of kin about what's going on and the management plan, etc.

'Trying to decide what to specialise in is tough! I loved surgery during medical school, hence why my foundation training is surgical-heavy – it's logical and varied, with theatre time, clinics and (short) ward rounds. I also like that it's fixing a problem in a tangible manner, e.g. a hemi-colectomy for colon cancer or a total hip replacement for a neck or femur fracture. Since working, I have come to appreciate the importance of work–life balance, so have veered away from the idea of surgery; I am now figuring out what would suit my work-needs better.

'I always come home feeling like I've achieved something – whether it's a correct diagnosis, being thanked by a next of kin for looking after a loved one, treating a septic patient or getting that tricky cannula in in one go! I like that every day is different – you never know what will happen when on call. I also love the steep learning curve – dealing with a sick patient on the wards and being that first port of call initially terrified me, however now it feels like second nature. I also appreciate that there is still more to learn; this job allows you to constantly progress, and that helps me stay interested. I never watch the clock when I'm working – the shifts go quickly!

'However, it is stressful, and every field of medicine has its own stresses. The long hours, the various shifts to adjust your sleeping pattern to and the constant bleeps. There can also be a sense of imposter syndrome.

'As for common "hot topics" that I actually deal with daily, these include sepsis and electrolyte imbalances like hypocalcaemia, hyperkalaemia and hyponatraemia. These are conditions that are increasingly impacting on patients that can be difficult to spot in the early stages.

'My advice to aspiring medics would be to make sure you really want to do it. I remember so many doctors discouraging me from applying during my work experience as a student. At the time it really irritated me because I thought it was a great career choice. Now that I am in it, I don't regret it, but I can appreciate why they felt jaded. It is a very long career path – the exams never end, the on-call shifts are tiring, patients will complain and the rate of burnout is high. So, maybe before applying, shadow a doctor while they're on call. Stay with them for the whole 13-hour shift and really put yourself in their shoes, because medicine is completely different once you've graduated and you're actually the one on call. My other tip would be to stay open-minded and see every opportunity in medicine as a learning opportunity. For example, if you go into a rotation/placement/work experience saying you hate surgery and want to be a GP, you won't get much out of it. However if you scrub into theatre and help assist, learn how to suture in the Emergency Department, ask questions when the team are reviewing x-rays, go to clinics and read around the subject, then you will gain so much from it and maybe even consider it as a speciality or at least take parts of what you learnt into your future speciality. We are privileged to get to learn about the human body, so enjoy it.'

2 | Work experience

Securing a formal work experience placement is not always a prerequisite for medical schools. However, undertaking work experience will undoubtedly bolster your application, while giving you an opportunity to reflect carefully on your decision to apply for medicine.

Why is work experience important?

Conducting work experience is typically an important part of your application: in doing work experience, you will be able to use your insights to communicate what it is about medicine that makes you want to pursue a career in the field, while being able to reflect on the less glamorous aspects of the job. It will also give you the opportunity to discuss your interests with doctors, which will allow you to garner a great deal of information about their working lives.

With this in mind, it is worth having these conversations with your own doctors, or even family and friends who work in the field of medicine. You could ask them about their time studying medicine at university and about the career options and prospects for those graduating in the field. Similarly, it is worth asking what their thoughts are on current issues and affairs in medicine and within the NHS. Remember to ask about the negative aspects as well as the positive; practising doctors are best placed to give you an accurate and honest answer.

Obtaining medical work experience can be difficult, so it is useful to get your applications in to local GP surgeries and hospitals in good time, as there can be waiting lists. Ask your school for support with obtaining work experience, as careers departments may have useful contacts.

Most work experience placements will involve shadowing a doctor. This is useful for a number of reasons:

- to help you in determining whether you really want to be a doctor
- to demonstrate your commitment to studying medicine
- to give you an insight into the varying nature of a doctor's working day, as well as their roles and responsibilities
- to provide good opportunities to discuss your interests in medicine
- if you make a good impression, you may be able to obtain a reference which your teacher can use to support your application.

How to arrange work experience

In some cases, your school will be able to support you by helping to organise work experience in the field of medicine, as they may have connections with local GP surgeries or hospitals. However, it is likely that only one work experience placement will be available through this route, so at some point in the process, you will need to show some initiative and organise some yourself. Where possible, you can try and utilise any contacts that your friends and family might have. The alternative approach is to contact local GP practices and hospitals to discuss the possibility of undertaking a placement.

To obtain a work experience placement, you should:

- research local practices or hospitals
- write a formal letter or email
- contact the appropriate department to identify the name of the person who will receive your letter – in hospitals, there is likely to be a dedicated individual in each area or ward who deals with these requests
- ask a teacher at your school if they will be your referee.

In addition, it is worth trying to secure placements in a medical environment, even if the role itself is not directly related to healthcare. Working on the reception desk in a GP surgery, for example, will still involve contact with patients and healthcare professionals, and can provide a valuable insight into their varying roles.

Example of a work experience request letter

Dear Mr Smith (*address the letter/email to the appropriate person*)

I would be very interested in applying for work experience at this hospital, and wondered whether any such opportunity might be available. I am currently in Year 12, studying for A levels in biology, chemistry and history, and would relish the chance to gain some practical experience during the forthcoming summer break.

I wondered whether it might be possible to meet with a doctor from your department to discuss the profession, and then perhaps spend a period of time shadowing one of your colleagues to obtain some first-hand experience.

If you require a reference, please contact my form tutor, Mr Jones, on mrjones@teacher.ac.uk.

Please do not hesitate to contact me if you require any further information or would like me to come to your office to meet you in person.

I look forward to hearing from you.

Yours sincerely,

Robert Smith

Things to look out for during your placement

As discussed, securing a work experience placement can be difficult, so it is crucial that you make the most of it while you are there. It will allow you to improve your understanding of medicine as a career, and will provide plenty of opportunities for you to reflect on the field for discussion later in your application. As such, you should pay close attention to what is going on around you.

You could make a good impression by:

- behaving impeccably at all times
- dressing formally
- asking questions to improve your understanding of a situation (however, you should also be aware of your surroundings; it may be insensitive to ask about a disease in front of a patient, or to ask complex questions while a doctor is carrying out a procedure)
- offering to help with routine tasks
- showing an interest in things that are going on around you.

There are several things that you should keep an eye out for when undertaking your work experience placement.

- **The attributes of a doctor.** Identify the key characteristics that they display, and most importantly, when they utilise them. In doing so, you will be able to identify the traits that you may need to develop.
- **How a doctor interacts with patients.** A key aspect of medicine is communication and, as discussed later in the book, it is likely to form a part of your application or be discussed at interview. You should pay close attention to how doctors deal with patients, including how they deliver news.
- **The tasks that the doctor carries out.** Again, this will give you an opportunity to see what kind of practical skills you might need to develop. It will give you an insight into the kind of things you might need to do yourself in several years' time.
- **The interventions carried out.** During your placement, you might see doctors prescribing drugs, conducting surgery or carrying out other medical procedures. Where necessary, you should consider asking what they are, and why they are being used. While you are not expected to understand the technical nature of medicine before studying it, these observations will enhance your understanding of the roles of a doctor from preventative to curative medicine.
- **The importance of a multidisciplinary team.** While your primary focus will probably be on the doctors, they do not function alone and rely heavily on other healthcare professionals, such as nurses, receptionists and administrators. If possible, you should also try and talk to these individuals, as it is important to develop your understanding of how a doctor is supported in their work.

You might also want to consider keeping a diary to write down what you see being done. This will allow you to conduct the most important aspect of carrying out work experience – reflection. At the time, you may think that you will remember what you saw, but it could be a long time between the work experience and an interview, and you will almost certainly forget vital details. Very often, applicants are asked at interview to expand on something interesting on their UCAS application. For example:

Interviewer: I see that you observed doctors treating a case of dystonia. What was that like?

Candidate: Er.

Interviewer: What exactly is dystonia? How was the patient treated?

Candidate: Um.

Don't allow this to happen to you!

A much better answer should go something like this …

Interviewer: I see that you observed doctors treating a case of dystonia. What was that like?

Candidate: Dystonia was not a condition that I had come across before, but it was immediately clear that it was a high pressure situation that needed to be resolved immediately due to the nature of the condition. This particular case was severe, and the patient's neck had been twisted to the side. He was in a great deal of discomfort.

Interviewer: What treatments are carried out for patients with these problems?

Candidate: In the emergency department, the patient was given a muscle relaxant to reduce the tension in the muscles and minimise the pain of the patient. This was not a recurrent situation for the patient and it was the first time he had experienced it, but the doctor was able to talk through the necessity for a referral to see a specialist neurologist. If the case can be put down to be an isolated incident, or not due to any particular disease, they might be treated with an injection of botulinum toxin directly into the affected muscles.

Interviewer: What is the botulinum toxin? Why would that be used?

Candidate: The botulinum toxin is produced by a type of bacteria known as Clostridium botulinum. The toxin blocks the release of the neurotransmitter acetylcholine at neuromuscular junctions. As a result, the muscle is unable to contract, which prevents dystonia.

Interviewer: What might the possible causative diseases be?

Candidate: My research has indicated that most commonly, the cause of dystonia remains unknown, though it is thought to be due to miscommunication between neurones in the brain. There are some neurodegenerative diseases, such as Parkinson's disease or multiple sclerosis, where dystonia is a symptom.

It can be difficult to persuade busy medical professionals to explain why they are carrying out each particular step. However, most will be willing to help, so time your questions accurately and approach members of the team who are most likely to provide you with the most insight.

Voluntary work

While work experience in a hospital or GP surgery is a useful way of identifying the key aspects of working as a doctor, it is also important to demonstrate your commitment to a career in medicine through more long-standing placements. Typically, these will be voluntary positions rather than work experience placements, and they will typically highlight the less glamorous aspects of a career in healthcare. A week spent helping elderly and confused patients walk to the toilet is worth a month in the hospital laboratory helping the technicians carry out routine tests.

Hospices and local care homes are usually happy to take on conscientious volunteers, and the work they do – caring for the terminally ill or the elderly – is particularly appropriate. Remember that you are not only working in these environments in order to learn about medicine in action. You are also there to prove, to yourself as well as to the admissions tutors, that you have the dedication and stomach for what is often an unpleasant and upsetting work environment. In completing work of this nature, you will be able to demonstrate your caring nature and develop your ability to deal with people.

TIP!

Because of health and safety regulations, it is not always possible to arrange work experience or voluntary work with GPs, in hospitals or in hospices. The medical schools' admissions tutors are aware of this but they will expect you to have found alternatives.

Voluntary work with a local charity is a good way of demonstrating your commitment as well as giving you the opportunity to find out more about medicine. The CEO of a leading charity confirmed this to us in a recent talk, when he said:

> *'The purpose of the voluntary sector is to help people in need. However, we need to help ourselves in order to survive as charities and continue to provide the support required by so many. Student volunteers are invaluable because they bring enthusiasm and purpose which the elderly respond to. While these work experiences are good for their applications to medical school, I would advise very strongly that they investigate the nature of the charity before they embark on it because work experience is only truly relevant and productive when you can connect to the work and the cause, not simply be undertaking it for the sake of ticking boxes.'*

Contact details for some of the respective charities can be found near the end of this book, although the list is by no means exhaustive.

It is important to note down key experiences while undertaking voluntary work. You should be sure to ask any questions that you might have and jot down the answers that you are given. It is also worth making a note of the dates and durations of your placements, as this will show that you are actually committed to working in a caring role, rather than merely completing placements to tick a box on your application form.

How work experience and voluntary work support your application

When you come to write the personal statement section of your UCAS application, you will need to reflect on your practical experience of medicine. While you will need to communicate what you did or what you observed, it is important not to simply list things. The admissions tutors will be looking for what you were able to take away from the experience in terms of what you learned about yourself, key aspects of a doctor's daily life and any attributes that they exhibited that made them good at their job. It is likely that some medical schools will question you about the contents of your personal statement, so it is important that you are able to talk in more depth about the points you mention.

For example, if you were to write: 'During the year that I worked on Sunday evenings at St Sebastian's Hospice, I saw a number of patients who were suffering from cancer and it was interesting to observe the treatment they received and watch its effects.' A generous interviewer will ask you about the management of cancer, and you have an opportunity to impress if you can explain the use of drugs, radiotherapy, diet, exercise, etc. The other benefit of work in a medical environment is that you may be able to make a good impression on the senior staff you have worked for. If they are prepared to write a brief reference and send it to your school, the teacher writing your reference will be able to quote from it.

Medical school admissions officers will be looking for an in-depth understanding of the medical profession, including what the career entails and the values and skills required to be a doctor. As well as talking to doctors and medical students, there are numerous online resources that will assist you in obtaining this knowledge. Free virtual medical work experience is now being provided by both Brighton and Sussex Medical School and the Royal College of General Practitioners. While they are not designed to replace face-to-face work experience entirely, completing these programmes can be really beneficial in supplementing your understanding and honing your application.

Virtual Work Experience Platform: Observe GP

Observe GP is a virtual learning experience for aspiring UK-based medics that provides an alternative to face-to-face work experience. The programme is organised by the Royal College of General Practitioners (RCGP) and supported by the Medical Schools Council. It is an interactive video platform that sets out to establish some of the realities of practising medicine as a GP, as well as the attributes required. It should take around 2.5 hours to complete, so it is worth looking into even if you have acquired face-to-face work experience!

More information can be found at www.rcgp.org.uk/your-career/work-experience/observe-gp.

Virtual Work Experience Platform: Brighton and Sussex Medical School

Brighton and Sussex Medical School recognised the importance of aspiring medical students gaining work experience, but also the limitations around accessing it for many people. As such, they set up their virtual work experience platform to give an insight into six medical specialities, including key attributes of the doctors and both the benefits and challenges of working within that speciality. The course should take up to 9 hours to complete.

More information can be found at https://bsmsoutreach.thinkific.com/courses/VWE.

Other things that you can do to support your application include the following.

- **Keep an eye on the news.** The NHS and illnesses that are badly impacting the UK feature on the news regularly, so it's easy to keep up with current events. Some media sources will put a political spin on their stories, so you will need to see past this and read from a variety of sources to get a balanced view.
- **Voluntary work.** There are plenty of voluntary opportunities worth exploring. The purpose of voluntary work is to gain an insight into care work, as well as learning about your own skills and attributes. You could explore whether any local community groups require support, or perhaps offer online opportunities, such as support groups. Nextdoor and Do-It.life are both organisations that coordinate voluntary work.
- **Independent learning.** Practising medicine involves a lifelong commitment to learning, so taking it upon yourself to learn something medicine-related can demonstrate that you are willing to do this. This can involve reading around topics of interest online, such as through the *British Medical Journal*'s open access information, listening to podcasts or watching relevant TED Talks. You could also complete an online course, such as those provided by FutureLearn (www.futurelearn.com), which usually run over a period of a few weeks.
- **Online resources and social media.** Beyond the virtual work experience platforms detailed on page 31, many student and junior doctors present their journeys through social media platforms such as YouTube and Instagram, as well as through blogs. While these are more informal, they can still provide a useful insight into the realities of medicine as a career.

The admissions officers and interviewers will also want to see that you understand the qualities required to succeed as a doctor, such as effective communication and being able to interact with a wide range of people. It would therefore be useful to consider the NHS Constitution, the details of which can be found here: www.gov.uk/government/publications/the-nhs-constitution-for-england.

3 | Deciding where to apply

Prior to submitting your application to medical school, it is essential that you conduct careful research into the application process, entrance requirements, the nature of the work that you will be conducting as a doctor, and the skills and traits that you will be required to demonstrate. If you have a thorough understanding of each of these aspects, your decision to study medicine will be a well-informed one and, for the most part, should improve your chances of gaining a place.

Choosing a medical school

Once you have made the decision to study medicine, you will need to carefully research medical schools. There are various factors that might influence your decision.

- The way that the course is delivered (such as whether the course is integrated, traditional, CBL, PBL or TBL).
- The academic (including GCSE and A level) requirements.
- The admissions tests that are required.
- The location of the university.
- The type of university.

You can obtain this information in a number of ways.

Online

A straightforward way of accessing information relating to the medical schools in the UK is using the UCAS website (www.ucas.com), which will often have links to the university websites too. It is important that you commit some time to exploring the information provided on both sites to find the information that you require. This information changes regularly, so if you are researching in advance, check back to make sure that nothing has changed closer to the time that you are submitting your application. If you are unable to get the answers you need from the internet, do not hesitate to contact the medical school either over the phone or via email.

An important point to note is that some medical schools offer more than one medicine course, including standard undergraduate degrees, postgraduate degrees and Foundation degrees. Make sure that you are looking at the appropriate course when conducting your research.

Open days

As well as researching medical schools online, you can also learn a great deal about them by visiting on open days. Information about open days can be obtained from university websites, or websites such as www.opendays.com. By attending an organised open day, you will be able to see the departments in which you will be studying and meet current academic staff and students, who will be able to answer any questions that you might have. You can also get a feel for the university in question – you will be spending the next five years of your life there, so it is important that you feel comfortable in that environment. If you don't, you might struggle to see the course through, irrespective of your academic achievements.

If you are planning on attending an open day, it is important that you ensure that you book onto any relevant talks to give yourself the best possible chance of obtaining the information that you need.

If you are unable to attend an organised open day, you should contact the university and ascertain whether there are any other opportunities to visit the department. In many cases, there will be someone who is able to meet you and give you a brief tour. If this is not possible, you can still visit on an informal basis to have a look around the university and see whether you like it, though you may not be able to visit the medical school itself.

Some universities also offer 'virtual open days', or opportunities to listen to talks from and speak with academic staff and students from specific university departments. A virtual open day is different to visiting a campus in person, yet still an excellent opportunity to see what a university has to offer and get an insight into a place where you might choose to study.

As you won't have to factor in travelling to the universities, you can attend more virtual open days than you might have initially intended, thus widening your options.

Virtual open days have differing formats depending on the university, but typically provide an opportunity to look at virtual tours, attend online webinars and talk to current students, lecturers and admissions officers, allowing you to ask any questions that you might have.

League tables

Another useful source of information regarding medical schools is university league tables, of which there are many available. The table below is compiled by the *Complete University Guide*, and bases its rankings on scores of student satisfaction, research quality and graduate prospects.

Table 2 Medical School rankings 2024

Medical school	Rank
University of Cambridge	1
University of Oxford	2
University of Glasgow	3
Imperial College London	4
University College London	5
University of Bristol	6
Queen's University Belfast	7
University of Edinburgh	8
University of Dundee	9
University of Leicester	10
Cardiff University	11
King's College London, University of London	12
Lancaster University	13
University of St Andrews	14
University of Sheffield	15
Queen Mary, University of London	16
Keele University	17
University of Aberdeen	18
University of Birmingham	19
University of Manchester	20
Hull York Medical School	21
University of Exeter	22
Newcastle University	23
University of East Anglia	24
University of Leeds	25
Brighton and Sussex Medical School	26
University of Liverpool	27
St George's, University of London	28
University of Nottingham	29
University of Southampton	30
University of Plymouth	31
University of Buckingham	32
University of Central Lancashire	33

Source: www.thecompleteuniversityguide.co.uk/league-tables/rankings/medicine. Reprinted with kind permission from the Complete University Guide *(www.thecompleteuniversityguide.co.uk).*

NB: League tables do not give a full picture and should be viewed only as one element of the decision-making process, rather than using it solely. In addition, different league tables use different information to rank medical schools, so it is worth looking into what exactly the positioning is based on. In reality, there is no bad medical school – all of those that deliver medicine degrees are approved by the General Medical Council.

MSC-approved medical schools

There are currently 41 medical schools or university departments of medicine in the UK that are recognised by the Medical Schools Council (MSC). These medical schools are summarised in Table 8 (pages 214–217). The London School of Hygiene and Tropical Medicine is also recognised by the MSC, but is not discussed here, since it provides only postgraduate qualifications in specific areas of medicine. Of these universities, the majority are accredited by the General Medical Council (GMC), while there are several schools in the UK currently under review. These schools include:

- Brunel Medical School
- University of Chester Medical School
- Edge Hill University Medical School
- Kent and Medway Medical School
- University of Sunderland School of Medicine
- Three Counties Medical School
- Ulster University School of Medicine.

For many of these medical schools, a number of restrictions applied to their first cohorts. It is always important to conduct research into any medical schools to which you are considering applying to ensure that there are no restrictions in place.

The University of Central Lancashire offers the majority of its places to international students, though a limited number of places are available to UK students resident in the north-west of England.

Brunel Medical School was newly established for 2021 entry, and runs a five-year undergraduate degree in medicine. In its first academic year, it was only open to international students, but applications for UK students are being considered from 2024.

The Three Counties Medical School at the University of Worcester is also recently established, and offers a graduate entry programme, with its first intake in September 2023. Currently, only students with a first degree are being considered, with priority given to those with substantial geographical links to the area (such as a childhood, parental or current address in the Three Counties area), Worcester graduates, first in the family to go to university, current resident in POLAR 1 and 2 quintiles, those working in the NHS (especially in the local area) and those with refugee status. The terms of entry may be expanded with changes to funding that may be available to the medical school in the future.

Similarly, the University of Surrey has also recently opened a medical school, with its first intake expected to be in February 2024. Applicants are only eligible if they are graduates, home students, and meet the requirements of the scholarships for UK students.

Ulster University School of Medicine is also open to graduates only at present, with its first intake in 2024.

While these universities are not yet accredited by the GMC, they are approved. Put simply, this means that the degrees obtained from these universities are not yet recognised for the practice of medicine in the UK, but this is standard for new medical schools; they do not become accredited until the first cohort has graduated. However, the GMC closely regulates the delivery of these degrees and annual reviews are available on the GMC website. You should not be put off by the lack of GMC accreditation of a medicine programme; in fact, each of the medical schools discussed above is guaranteed by an established medical school, meaning that if anything were to go wrong, you would graduate from the guarantor medical school instead.

The University of Buckingham, a privately funded university, is recognised by the MSC. It was added to the GMC's accredited list of universities in May 2019 following the graduation of its first cohort of students. Swansea University, Warwick Medical School and Ulster Medical School also appear on the MSC list, although they only offer Graduate Entry (A101) programmes.

The universities on the list offer a range of options for students wishing to study medicine:

- five- or six-year MBBS or MBChB courses (UCAS codes A100 or A106)
- four-year accelerated graduate-entry courses (A101, A102 or A109)
- six-year courses that include a 'pre-med' year (A103 or A104).

Entry requirements of all medical schools are also summarised in Table 8 (pages 214–217).

Factors to consider when choosing a medical school

You can apply to up to four medical schools in one application cycle. In deciding which to eliminate, you may find the following points helpful.

- **Grades and retakes.** If you are worried that you will not achieve a minimum of three A grades at A level the first time round, it is worth doing some careful research into which universities consider retake candidates (see Table 8, pages 214–217). While there is an increasing number of medical schools that will consider students who are retaking their A levels, some will only consider your application a second time if you applied to them in the first instance, or if you secured particular grades the first time around.
- **Interviews.** All medical schools interview A level candidates; some still use traditional panel interviews, while the majority use Multiple Mini Interviews (MMIs). Each school's interview policy is shown in Table 9 (see pages 218–220).
- **Location and socialising.** You may be attracted to the idea of being at a campus university rather than at one of the medical schools that are not located on the campuses of their affiliated universities. One reason for this may be that you would like to mix with students from a wide variety of disciplines and that you will enjoy the intellectual and social cross-fertilisation. However, it is worth keeping in mind that medical school hours and demands are arduous, so identifying a university solely based on opportunities for socialising is not advised!
- **Course structure.** While all the medical schools are well equipped and provide a high standard of teaching, there are real differences in the way the courses are taught and examined and you will not find two the same. Specifically, the majority offer an integrated course in which students see patients at an early stage and certainly before the formal clinical part of the course. The other main distinction is between systems-based courses (e.g. Manchester and Liverpool), which teach medicine in terms of the body's systems (e.g. the cardiovascular system), and subject-based courses (e.g. Oxford and Cambridge), which teach in terms of the fundamental subjects (anatomy, biochemistry, etc.).
- **Teaching style.** The style of teaching can also vary from place to place. See pages 8–19 for more information on PBL, CBL, TBL, integrated and traditional approaches to teaching.
- **Intercalated degrees and electives.** Another difference in the courses offered are the opportunities for an intercalated Honours degree and electives. The intercalated degree scheme allows students to tack on one further year of study either to the end of the two-year pre-clinical course or as an integrated part of a six-year course. Successful completion of this year, which may be used to study a wide variety of subjects, confers an Honours degree qualification. Electives

are periods of work experience away from the medical school and, in some cases, abroad. See pages 19–21 for more information.

Academic requirements

By the time you read this you will probably have chosen your GCSE subjects or even taken them. If not, here are some points to consider.

- While there are obviously exceptions, most universities specify particular grades (typically A/7 or B/6) in English language, maths and science subjects (whether dual, triple or core and additional). You will need to carefully research the requirements for each medical school and ensure that you meet the requirements before applying there. Many medical schools ask for a 'good' set of GCSE results. What this means exactly varies considerably from university to university, but on average, a minimum of five GCSEs at grade A/7 or B/6, including the aforementioned core subjects.
- Most medical schools require the study of chemistry, plus at least one other science (biology or physics) or maths. For the most part, the second science subject requested is usually biology. However, there is an increasing amount of flexibility with subject choices, with a number of universities no longer stating chemistry as an A level requirement. At the time of writing, these universities include Anglia Ruskin, East Anglia, Keele, Kent, Lancaster, Leeds, Leicester, Manchester, Newcastle, Plymouth, Queen Mary, Sheffield, Southampton and Sunderland, though it is important to closely check university websites at the time.
- If AS level examinations are completed, these are likely to be taken into account by the admissions tutors reviewing your application. If it is your school's policy to sit these exams in year 12, it is important to remember that they are stand-alone qualifications and should therefore be taken seriously.

If you have already taken your GCSEs and achieved disappointing grades, carefully research the GCSE requirements of each university and identify those where you have the best possible chance. If it is genuinely the case, your referee can vouch for you and indicate in your reference that your A level attainment is unlikely to be a reflection of your GCSE performance. To prove this is the case, it is crucial that you work extremely hard for your A levels.

In the case of mitigating circumstances that have impacted your attainment at GCSE, you should contact the university admissions department to ascertain what the required procedure is in that situation. For the most part, a comment from your teacher in your reference will be sufficient, but they may also require a separate form or letter including evidence of the circumstances before they will consider your application.

AS levels

Given that the policy for most schools is that AS level examinations are not compulsory, the general stance for medical schools is that AS grades will no longer be part of any offers made and they do not have an explicit AS grade requirement. However, Queen's University Belfast will judge a candidate's application on whether they have been able to sit a fourth AS exam at their school, in that their standard offer is AAA plus an A grade in a fourth subject at AS level. However, concessions can be made to this, and if the AS level cannot be provided, the offer is increased to A*AA or A*A*A dependent on subject choices.

If AS levels are included in the application, they will serve as a reasonable indicator of anticipated attainment overall, so it is likely that admissions tutors may consider them. As such, it is crucially important that you work hard from the start of the course so that you are thoroughly prepared for AS examinations, as they will form a part of your application, even though they do not contribute to your overall A level grade.

A level choices

Your choice of A levels

You will see from Table 8 (pages 214–217) that, with the exception of Newcastle University, all medical schools now ask for just two science/maths subjects at A level. When choosing your A level subjects, there are three important considerations.

1. Choose subjects that you are good at. You must be capable of an A grade as a minimum requirement. If you aren't sure, ask your teachers.
2. Choose subjects that will help you in your medical course; life at medical school is tough enough as it is without having to learn new subjects from scratch.
3. It is wholly acceptable to choose a non-scientific third subject that you enjoy and that will provide you with an interesting topic of conversation at your interview. With the exception of general studies, critical thinking and, in many cases, further maths, universities do not discriminate based on the third subject. Students who can cope with the differing demands of arts and sciences at A level have an advantage in that they can demonstrate breadth.

So what combination of subjects should you choose? In addition to chemistry/biology and another science at A level, you might also consider subjects such as psychology, sociology or a language. Psychology as a subject has become more mathematical, as well as scientific; as such, Edge Hill University, Keele University, the Kent and Medway Medical School, Lancaster University, the University of Leicester, the University of Manchester, Plymouth University and the University of Sheffield will now regard it as a second science subject in their grade offers. The point to bear in mind when you are making your choices is that you need high grades, so do not pick a subject that sounds interesting, such as Italian, if you are not good at languages. Similarly, although an A level in further maths might look good on your UCAS application, you will need to consider if it is actually something universities want you to have. You will need to check the individual requirements; most medical schools will indicate preferred A level subjects in addition to science A levels.

Taking four A levels

There's no harm in doing more than three A levels (and an AS exam, if offered by your school), but there is really no advantage to it. In most cases, the added pressure of studying for a fourth A level means that you run the risk of pulling down your overall grades, so you might consider dropping the additional qualification at the end of year 12. Medical schools will not include the fourth A level in any conditional offers they make.

If you are taking the International Baccalaureate, then you should still be aiming to take biology and chemistry, as these are the subjects required for undergraduate study. However, some universities specify chemistry and one of maths, biology, human biology and physics. If you are not taking these subjects, you should be considering what makes you think you will be able to cope on a medicine course. For Scottish students, you are expected to have at least two Advanced Highers and three Highers, with biology and chemistry and usually either maths or physics as well to at least Higher level; Imperial College, for example, asks for five Highers and three Advanced Highers to A grade standard. Overall, students should be aiming for majority A grades in Highers and Advanced Highers, though AB at Advanced Highers is accepted, or even BB in the case of the University of Edinburgh, for example.

The prediction

The admissions tutor will look for a grade prediction in the reference that your teacher writes about you. Your teacher will make a prediction based on the reports of your subject teachers, your GCSE grades and, most importantly, the results of any exams taken at the end of year 12.

Consequently, it is vital that you work hard during the first year of A levels. Only by doing so will you get the reference you need. If there is any reason or excuse to explain why you did badly at GCSE or did not work hard in year 12, you must make sure that the teacher writing your reference knows about it and includes it in the reference. The most common reasons for poor performance are illness and problems at home (e.g. illness of a close relation or family breakdown). In many cases, additional evidence will be required by the university to support this claim, so stating that you underperformed due to ill health when this is not the case is likely to cause bigger problems.

The bottom line is that you need to persuade your school that you are on track for grades of AAA or higher, depending on where you are applying. Convincing everyone else usually involves convincing yourself!

Non-medical choices

Although you can apply to a total of five institutions through UCAS, you may apply to only four medical schools. What should you do with the final slot? Applying for an alternative, non-medical course will not jeopardise your medicine application in any way, but the fifth choice is still worthy of careful consideration for a number of reasons. There are two main options regarding the fifth choice.

1. Do not include a fifth choice

If you are truly committed to becoming a doctor, you need to consider whether you would realistically accept your fifth choice course. If you know that you would not consider that course in place of medicine and would prefer to reapply, it may be in your best interests to leave the final choice blank. If you were then unfortunate enough to not secure a place to study medicine, you could spend a year developing your application in order to boost your chances the following academic year.

2. Carefully consider an alternative course

You might choose to include a non-medical choice on your form if you are not prepared to wait for a year if your application is unsuccessful, or if you intend to enter medicine as a graduate (see below).

Trying to combine two different subjects in your personal statements is a recipe for disaster. While admissions tutors cannot see which other courses you have applied for on your UCAS application, it will automatically signal to both departments that you are not really committed to either course. This would be especially apparent if you were including a subject such as chemical engineering or archaeology as your fifth choice. As such, under no circumstances should this be done; simply stick to medicine with the personal statement in your UCAS application.

If there is a course that you would genuinely consider studying in place of medicine, or perhaps you are already reapplying and just want to go to university next academic year, there are ways of applying to two separate courses. For the most part, students will want to apply to another science-based course, which minimises the problems associated with the personal statement. However, it does not completely eradicate them.

If you do intend to include a fifth choice which you would genuinely consider in the case of an unsuccessful medicine application, then you may need to contact the university in question to ascertain whether or not they will consider this application. Many universities will happily consider this option once you have contacted them to explain why your personal statement does not match up with the course, but some may request an additional personal statement. In this case, you must be prepared to deliver a second personal statement outlining why you are committed to studying that course if you are to successfully acquire a place. This is becoming especially common where students choose other vocational degrees, such as pharmacy or optometry, as their back-up choices.

Many students now pursue the option of undertaking a first degree in a related subject, such as biomedical science, which they then utilise as a platform to gain access onto medicine as a second degree.

To BSc ... or not to BSc?

As discussed above, many students who are initially unsuccessful in their pursuit of medicine will undertake a related science degree first, such as biomedical science or biochemistry. Whether or not to consider a BSc in lieu of a medicine degree is a very tricky question, but ultimately, it can be answered by no one other than you. There are several pros and cons worth considering.

Cons

- You might spend a whole three years on a course you never really wanted to study. Studying a subject at degree level is an enormous commitment, and if you are not entirely motivated by the content, it can be a very trying time.
- Three years of study will add additional cost and time before actually getting into medical school.
- Entry to medical school after graduating is not guaranteed.
- If admitted to undergraduate medical school only, you will still have to study for five more years.
- You might lose focus on medicine if you study something else first.
- You may not get the student funding and help towards fees, compared with if you go straight after A levels.

Pros

- Many BSc degrees are in biomedical or medical subjects – if you wouldn't enjoy these, would you enjoy medicine, which is not that different?
- Medicine is a lifelong commitment, so two to three years of additional study should not worry you. Becoming a good doctor is a journey, not a target.
- Although entry to medical school is not guaranteed, some BSc courses do offer a very secure pathway to overseas medical schools in the event you don't get in to one in the UK.
- Applying as a graduate certainly makes your medical school application stronger as you have matured as an individual and academically.

- Having a BSc as well as a medical degree may enhance your chances to get the medical job you desire – a reason why many medical students intercalate.
- Studying a first degree will give you time to mature as a person. You will become acquainted with the demands of university life and develop your skills in independent study. Many students who take this approach find that by the time they reach medical school, they are more comfortable with the workload and can approach the study of medicine with greater confidence.

Applying to Oxbridge medical schools

Oxbridge is in a separate category because, if getting into most medical schools is difficult, entry into Oxford or Cambridge is even more so (the extra hurdles facing students wishing to apply to Oxford or Cambridge are discussed in *Getting into Oxford & Cambridge*, another guide in this series). The general advice given here also applies to Oxbridge, but the competition is intense, and before you include either university on your UCAS application you need to be confident that you can achieve the entrance standard grades (A*A*A at Cambridge and A*AA at Oxford) at A level and that you will interview well.

You cannot apply to both Oxford and Cambridge in your application and your teachers will advise you whether to apply to either. You should discuss an application to Oxford or Cambridge with your teachers at an early stage. You would need a good reason to apply to Oxbridge against the advice of your teachers and it certainly is not worth applying on the 'off chance' of getting in. By doing so you will simply waste one of your valuable four choices.

When considering an Oxbridge application, you must carefully consider which of the two universities you will apply to, and in addition, the college at which you are interested in studying. There is no disadvantage to submitting an open application, which means that each college can consider your application and invite you to interview. An important distinction between Oxford and Cambridge and other universities is their tutorial system. You will meet with a tutor, alongside two or three other medicine students from your college, to discuss a particular topic in great depth. These sessions are often accompanied by a significant amount of work specific to each college.

Both Oxford and Cambridge will be looking for all of the attributes in your application that show that you will make an outstanding doctor. It is also worth remembering, however, that the elite universities are highly academic, so it may be worth adding in a little extra in your applications. This may be associated with areas of research that interest you, or wider reading that you have conducted in specific areas of medicine.

4 | The UCAS application

There are various components to a medicine application that will ultimately determine whether or not you are made an offer. The first component of the application to study medicine in the UK is completion of the UCAS application form. Some sections of the application are purely factual, such as your name, address and prior examination results, as well as a section where you enter your choice of medical schools. Perhaps most importantly, you must include a personal statement, which gives you an opportunity to write about why you want to study medicine and what would make you a good fit for the course and career. In addition, a teacher will provide a reference which supports your application.

The application is critical, as this is what the admissions tutors at each university that you apply to will receive. On reviewing your application, the admissions tutors will make a decision as to whether or not you will be invited to interview. With the exception of one UK medical school, you will need to attend a face-to-face interview in order to gain a conditional offer.

What happens to your application

By the October deadline, medical schools will have received an extremely high number of applications which far exceeds the number of places that they have. Some UK medical schools can receive up to almost ten times as many applications as they have places, which admissions tutors will then review to ascertain who deserves the opportunity to prove themselves at interview. Admissions tutors have the ruthless task of culling applications that are insufficient, and painstakingly reviewing those that remain.

Most medical schools have a well-defined set of criteria which students should consider before submitting an application. Typically, the first part of the selection process by admissions tutors will be ruling out any applicant who does not meet these criteria in full, so it is crucial that you take the time to check that you do meet the criteria. The majority of admissions tutors are happy to discuss these aspects of the application with you, so make sure that you conduct your research in good time and where necessary, get in touch with them to see whether you are eligible.

For the most part, students applying to medicine will have been predicted the required grades (which are typically AAA or higher), or in some circumstances, may have obtained them already. In addition, a high proportion of applicants will have a good set of GCSE or equivalent results. The academic demands are consistently high with medicine, so it is unlikely that academic attainment alone will be sufficient to make your application stand out.

This is where the rest of your application comes in, and in particular, your personal statement and academic reference. The personal statement should discuss your motivation to study medicine, as well as your work experience or voluntary work and what undertaking it has taught you about working in this particular healthcare setting. Your reference, usually provided by a teacher at your school, will then discuss your strengths as a student.

In order to decide whom to call for interview, the admissions tutors will have to make a decision based solely on the information presented to them. If your application does not demonstrate the necessary requirements at this stage, irrespective of how outstanding your personal qualities are, you will not be invited to interview, which means that the university in question cannot make you an offer.

The sample medical interview selection form opposite gives an example of the ways in which your application might be viewed by admissions tutors. When preparing to apply, it might be worth you using this as a rough way of assessing your own application, and identifying ways in which you could strengthen it.

The UCAS form

The online UCAS form is accessed through the UCAS website (www. ucas.com). Applicants will need to generate an account on the UCAS Hub. The UCAS Hub is a free tool that allows you to conduct research into your options beyond sixth form and store it all in an accessible way, as well as providing useful resources to help with personal statement and CV writing. Previously, the UCAS Hub and UCAS Apply registrations were separate, with different login information; UCAS has combined the two to eliminate confusion. While it is encouraged that you utilise the UCAS Hub fully, as it is an excellent resource, you can just use it to create an account for your application.

Upon generating an account, you will be asked for the year of entry, the level of study that you are interested in, the country that you are from, your contact preferences and subject areas of interest. These answers

MEDICAL INTERVIEW SELECTION FORM		
Name: Age at entry: Selector:	UCAS number: Gap year?: Date:	
SELECTION CRITERIA COMMENTS		
1 Academic (score out of 10) GCSE results/AS grades/A level predictions UCAT/BMAT result 2 Commitment (score out of 10) Genuine interest in medicine? Relevant work experience? Community involvement? 3 Personal (score out of 10) Range of interests? Involvement in school activities? Achievements and/or leadership? Referee supports application?		
Total score (maximum of 30):		
Recommendation of selector:	Interview Reserve list Rejection	Score 25–30 Score 16–24 Score 0–15
Further comments (if any):		

Figure 3 Sample candidate selection form

will tailor the information presented to you on the UCAS Hub. Most applicants register through their school or college using the institution's buzzword, but it is possible to register independently. Once the account has been created, you can access the UCAS form through the applications section. The application sections are summarised below:

- Profile: upon creating an account you will be asked to fill in your personal details, including funding and sponsorship options, residential status, details of any criminal convictions, and the individual selected as your nominated access (someone who can talk to UCAS on your behalf if required). The 'more about you' section is new to the application form for 2023, and allows you to disclose any circumstances for which you might need support during your studies, such as special educational needs or a disability.

- Experience: this section covers your education and employment histories and extra activities. For the education section, you will need to add in any qualifications that you hold with the grade obtained; and for qualifications you are currently studying, with the grade left as 'pending'. In the employment section you can add in the details of paid jobs. The extra activities section allows you to include the details of activities you have taken part in to prepare for higher education, such as summer schools, taster courses, booster courses, university-led programmes or regional and national schemes.
- Personal statement: you will need to write a personal statement that outlines your motivation for studying the course that you have applied for with a limit of 4,000 characters and 47 lines; this will be reviewed by admissions tutors.
- Course choices: in this section, you can add in up to five university or college choices. Remember that for medical school you can only add four choices; with your fifth choice you can put down an alternative course, but this is not obligatory. If you are applying for deferred entry, you can choose this option here.
- Reference: once you have completed your application, you will click send. If you are applying through your school or college, the application will first be sent to that institution, which will check your application and submit your reference. This means that your form can get returned to you at this point if there are any mistakes that need correcting. If you are applying independently, you will be asked for the details of a referee, who will then be contacted by email and asked to upload a reference before you are able to send your application to UCAS. Your reference is usually provided by a teacher, or someone who knows you professionally.

Despite the help that spelling- and grammar-check programs can provide, it is still possible to create an unfavourable impression on the admissions tutors through spelling mistakes, grammatical errors and unclear personal statements. In order to ensure that this does not happen, follow these tips.

- Read the instructions for each section of the application carefully before filling it in.
- Double-check all dates (when you joined and left schools, when you sat examinations), examination boards, GCSE grades and personal details (fee codes, residential status codes, disability codes).

- Plan your personal statement as you would an essay. Lay it out in a logical order. Make the sentences short and to the point. Split the section into paragraphs, covering each of the necessary topics (i.e. reasons for wanting to study medicine, work experience and voluntary work, academic interests and extracurricular activities and achievements). This will enable the selectors to read and assess it quickly and easily.
- Ask your teachers to cast a critical eye over your draft, and don't be too proud to make changes in the light of their advice.

Once your application has been submitted, you can keep track of the responses from the universities using UCAS Track.

Timing

The main UCAS submission period is from early September to the end of January, but medical applications have to be with UCAS by mid-October, typically on the closest weekday to 15 October. Late applications are also permitted, although medical schools are not bound to consider them. Remember that most referees take at least a week to consult the relevant teachers and compile a reference, so allow for that and aim to submit your application by mid-September unless there is a good reason for delaying.

The only convincing reason for delaying is that your teachers cannot predict high A level grades at the moment, but might be able to do so if they see high-quality work during the autumn term. If you are not being predicted the minimum grades required, it does not necessarily mean that you won't be able to apply, but it will require some careful research and contact with admissions tutors to establish whether or not you would be considered.

Interviews usually take place between November and March of the academic year and so if you have not heard by January, it is not necessarily a negative situation.

The reference

The reference will be written by a referee who could be your headteacher, housemaster, personal tutor or head of sixth form. They will write about what an outstanding person you are and about your contribution to school life as well as your academic achievement (i.e. on target for at least three A grades at A level), and they will then also give reasons why you are suitable to study medicine. For them to say this it must of course be true, as referees have to be as honest as possible and they will accurately assess your character and potential to succeed at university. You must have demonstrated to your teachers and other members of staff that you have all the necessary qualities required to become a doctor.

Ideally, your efforts to impress them will have begun at the start of the sixth form (or preferably before this); you will have become involved in school activities, while at the same time working hard on your A level subjects and developing strong interpersonal skills, demonstrated by your interactions with staff and students. If you do not feel as though you have done this, don't worry, because it is never too late. Some people mature later than others, so if this does not sound like you, start to make efforts to get involved in the wider life of your school or college, as this will help provide evidence for the people who will contribute to your reference.

To what extent does your referee support your application?

It is vitally important to make sure that your referee knows all about your work experience in hospitals and in the local community. Remember that the teacher writing your reference will rely heavily on advice from other teachers too. You can help yourself by working hard, looking keen and talking about medicine, where relevant, in class. Ask questions that display your genuine interest in becoming a doctor or a particular topic, as well as thinking beyond the confines of the syllabus in class and ask intelligent, medicine-related questions such as those given below. Do not try and ask complicated medical questions for the sake of it; ask questions because you genuinely wish to know the answer and could carry on the conversation once given the answer.

- How effective is gene therapy in the treatment of cystic fibrosis?
- How does being obese actually contribute to suffering from type 2 diabetes?
- Is it because enzymes become denatured at over 45°C that patients suffering from heatstroke have to be cooled down quickly using ice?
- Could sex-linked diseases such as muscular dystrophy be avoided by screening the sperm to eliminate those containing the X chromosomes that carry the harmful recessive genes from an affected male?

As part of the reference your referee will need to predict the grades that you are likely to achieve. The entry requirements of the medical schools are shown in Table 8 (pages 214–217). If you are predicted lower than the requirements it is almost certain that you will not be considered. Talk to your teachers and find out whether you are on target for these grades. If not, you may need to work harder to show them what you're capable of, or you may want to hold back on your application until you have achieved your grades.

If you are a mature student or going through graduate entry, the referee could be a lecturer from your university who will provide the appropriate information.

The UCAS reference form is divided into three sections. The first section allows your referee to include background information about the school or centre itself, including context such as performance, intake demographics and rates of progression to higher education. It also allows referees to explain any restrictions of subject provisions, information about the school that may have impacted performance (such as changes to staffing or damage to buildings), and approaches to predicting grades (such as the internal assessments used) – this will often be the same for every individual at the centre. If you are applying independently, this section allows the referee to outline their professional relationship to you. The second section will be filled in by your referee if it is applicable, as it provides the opportunity to give any information regarding possible extenuating circumstances that contextualise the academic journey of the applicant, such as illness, bereavement, adverse personal circumstances or being a mature student. In this section, your referee can discuss any disparity between predicted grades and attained grades, subject choices if they have differed from those requested, and any additional support that has been provided that would also be beneficial at university level. The third and final section is where the referee provides evidence of suitability of the applicant to the course, including academic and extracurricular achievements, work experience, voluntary work, etc.

What happens next and what to do about it

Once your reference has been written and the overall application submitted, a receipt will be sent to your school or college to acknowledge its arrival. Your application is then processed and UCAS will send you confirmation of your details. If you don't receive this, you should check with your referee that it has been correctly submitted. The confirmation will contain your application number, your details and the list of courses to which you have applied.

Check carefully to make sure that the details in your application have been saved to the UCAS system correctly. At the same time, make a note of your UCAS number – you will need to quote this when you contact the medical schools.

Now comes a period of waiting, which can be very unsettling but which must not distract you from your studies. Most medical schools decide whether or not they want to interview you within a few months.

- If one or more of the medical schools decides to interview you, your next letter will be an invitation to visit the school and attend an interview. (For advice on how to prepare for the interview, see Chapter 6.)

- If you are unlucky, the next correspondence you get from UCAS will contain the news that you have been rejected by one or more of your chosen schools. Does a rejection mean it's time to relax on the A level work and dust off alternative plans? Should you be reading up on exactly what the four-year course in road resurfacing involves? No, you should not!

A rejection is a setback and it does make the path into medicine that bit steeper, but it isn't an excuse to give up. A rejection should act as a spur to work even harder because the grades you achieve at A level are now even more important. Don't give up and do turn to Chapter 8 to see what to do when you get your A level results.

Deferral of place

If you are going to apply to study medicine, you should expect to start as soon as possible, unless, and this is important, there is a good reason for you to make a deferral request. Bear in mind, universities are under no pressure to defer places as they put greater emphasis on places available for first-time applicants, except in extenuating circumstances. However, they do have roughly a 10% quota of students annually who will defer their places and they are sometimes happy to grant these requests if the student can prove they will be doing something worthwhile with their gap year. If there is a compelling reason, talk it through with them first to discuss your options.

Case study

Anushka is a fourth-year medical student at Lancaster University.

'My curiosity of the functioning of the human body, coupled with the rapidly evolving nature of medicine initiated my interest in becoming a doctor. Illnesses that were thought to be incurable are now being cured due to new discoveries being made. It is this that motivated me to pursue a career in medicine.

'Before applying to study medicine, I volunteered at my local care home and the British Heart Foundation charity shop. My main role at the care home was to help feed the residents, however I tried to be as involved as possible in all care needs of the residents. Work experience built my confidence and enhanced my communication skills. These key skills form the foundations of a doctor, and is something you can build as you progress in your career. In my opinion, the earlier you get exposure and experience in these skills, the better.

'Unfortunately, I did not achieve my A level grades that were required for entrance into medical school first time around. Enrolling at MPW was the best decision I have ever made. With their expertise and support, I was able to achieve my predicted grades in Biology, Chemistry and Mathematics of A*AA and get offers from two medical schools.

'I am thoroughly enjoying my time at medical school. Although it can be challenging at times, due to the vast quantity of work, once you establish your studying technique, you begin to appreciate your theoretical knowledge and clinical practice. It is rewarding to see conditions you have studied be treated when you attend placement in hospital.

'My medical school incorporates professional ethics into the medical course. I really enjoy this aspect as we have ethical case debates every year, in which doctors and students can participate.

'Medicine is an extensive subject, where it is impossible to know everything, yet difficult to ascertain how much depth is enough for your level. This can sometimes get quite overwhelming, and you may find yourself with little flexibility in your work–life balance.

'Although I am unsure of the particular speciality I want to pursue in my career, within 10 years I would want to be in my speciality training, and potentially close to becoming a consultant.

'My top three tips for prospective medical students would be:

- Get work experience as early as possible in care homes, charity shops, GPs, etc.
- Make sure that you thoroughly prepare for interviews, with mock interviews at your school if possible.
- Do plenty of practice for your UCAT and BMAT entrance exams.'

Aptitude tests

Almost all UK medical schools ask applicants to sit aptitude tests as part of the application process. At undergraduate level, these tests include either the UCAT or the BMAT tests.

UCAT (University Clinical Aptitude Test)

The UCAT has been adopted by 36 universities in the UK as part of their admissions procedures, and helps them make an informed choice between the highest-performing candidates for undergraduate medical study. It is designed to ensure that students have the mental capabilities, attitude and professional conduct required for a medical career. It is not a test of your curriculum knowledge or any scientific background. The UCAT tests thought processes and as such cannot be revised for, though it is possible to prepare yourself in order to boost your overall attainment.

The UCAT is a computer-based test, and this aspect of the test should not be underestimated: your eyes will get very tired after staring at a computer screen for two hours, so make sure that at least some of your preparation is done online.

The UCAT must be completed at an official Pearson VUE test centre. Test centres can be found in many locations worldwide, so identify which test centres are local to you. If there is a problem with you attending any of these test centres, consult the UCAT website (www.ucat.ac.uk).

Registration is typically open between May and September and the test is sat between early July and the end of September, though the earlier you take it, the better. By reserving an early slot, you will be able to sit the UCAT with a clear head, and it will give you more time to research which universities will consider your overall application, inclusive of the UCAT score. In addition, if you become unwell or are unable to make your booked test for any reason, you have the opportunity to reschedule for a later date. If you book your initial test too late in the cycle, then it is unlikely that there will be local slots remaining for you to complete it, meaning that you have to sit the test when you're ill or travel a considerable distance to take it! However, you must also ensure that you have given yourself sufficient time to prepare for the test, so you will need to try and strike a balance with the test date that you opt for.

If you have any disabilities or additional needs that require you to have extra time in examinations, it is important that you register for the UCATSEN instead of the regular test. For example, if you require 25% additional time in examinations due to a diagnosis of dyslexia, the UCATSEN will allocate this additional time to each section of the exam. If you require special access arrangements for examinations, then you should directly contact Pearson VUE customer services to discuss these arrangements before you book the test.

There are five separately timed sections to the UCAT. These sections are based on a set of skills that medical (and dental) schools believe are vital to be successful as a medical practitioner.

1. **Verbal Reasoning.** Candidates are provided with a piece of text that they have to analyse and answer questions on. This section assesses the ability of the candidate to critically evaluate written information.
2. **Decision Making.** This test assesses a candidate's ability to apply logic to reach a decision or conclusion, evaluate arguments and analyse statistical information.
3. **Quantitative Reasoning.** This section assesses a candidate's ability to critically evaluate information presented in a numerical form.
4. **Abstract Reasoning.** Candidates are presented with a series of shapes that they must interpret and identify patterns within. This section assesses the use of convergent and divergent thinking to infer relationships.

5. **Situational Judgement.** This tests candidates' ability to comprehend real-world situations and to identify critical factors and appropriate behaviour in handling them.

The test lasts two hours in total. Those candidates with special educational needs take the UCATSEN and are given the allocated additional time per section.

Table 3 Timings for UCAT/UCATSEN

Section	Items	Standard Test Time	Extra Time/ UCATSEN
Verbal Reasoning	44 items	22 minutes	27.5 minutes
Decision Making	29 items	32 minutes	40 minutes
Quantitative Reasoning	36 items	25 minutes	31.25 minutes
Abstract Reasoning	55 items	14 minutes	17.25 minutes
Situational Judgement	69 items	27 minutes	33.75 minutes
Total time		120 minutes	150 minutes

Dates

A list of important dates regarding the UCAT exam can be found at www.ucat.ac.uk. For reference, the key dates for 2024 were:

- UCAT account creation opens: 14 May
- test booking begins: 18 June
- testing begins: 8 July
- account creation and booking closes: 19 September (12 noon)
- last testing date: 26 September

Please check the UCAT website for updates.

Universities that require the UCAT

Table 4 (below) shows the UK universities that require students to sit the UCAT as part of their application process.

Table 4 Medical schools requiring UCAT admissions test

Medical school	UCAS course code
University of Aberdeen	A100, A105
Anglia Ruskin University	A100
Aston University	A100
University of Birmingham	A100, A101
University of Bristol	A100, A108
Brunel University	A100
Cardiff University	A100, A104

University of Central Lancashire	A100
University of Chester	A101
University of Dundee	A100, A104
University of East Anglia	A100, A104
Edge Hill University	A100, A110
University of Edinburgh	A100
University of Exeter	A100
University of Glasgow	A100
Hull York Medical School	A100, A101
Keele University	A100, A104
Kent and Medway Medical School	A100
King's College London	A100, A101, A102
University of Leeds	A100, A101
University of Leicester	A100, A199
University of Liverpool	A100
University of Manchester	A101, A104, A106
Newcastle University	A100, A101
University of Nottingham	A100, A10L, A108, A18L
University of Plymouth (Peninsula Schools of Medicine and Dentistry)	A100
Queen Mary University of London	A100, A101, A110
Queen's University Belfast	A100
University of Sheffield	A100, A101, A102
University of Southampton	A100, A101, A102
University of St Andrews	A100, A990
St George's, University of London	A100
University of Sunderland	A100
University of Surrey	A101
University of Warwick	A101
University of Worcester	A101

Preparation

Although the UCAT website tries to discourage students from doing any preparation for the test other than sitting the practice tests available online, students who have sat the test in the past have found that the more practice they had on timed IQ-type tests, the better prepared they felt. In this chapter you will find practice questions for each section.

General hints

- Use the practice questions provided on the following pages to familiarise yourself with the type of questions that are asked and the time constraints in the test. It is important to practise the different types of question available so that you can improve your approach to each question type.

- Most candidates have great difficulty completing the sections of the test in the allocated time, so don't panic if you find that this is the case when you are practising questions. The UCAT website provides practice tests that can be completed online, and these give a realistic representation of the level of questioning you will get in the official exam, as well as the timing and the practical aspects of completing tests on a computer.
- There is a point for each right answer, but no points are deducted for wrong answers.
- Try not to leave blanks. If you really can't work out the answer, it is better to eliminate the answers that you know to be wrong and then make your best guess from those that are left. The answers are multiple-choice and, as the test is not negatively marked, it is better to have a go!
- Throughout the test, there is an option to 'flag' questions. If you are struggling with a question, it is best to have a guess at an answer, flag the question and move on. Then, providing you have time remaining at the end, you can easily identify which questions to return to so that you can work through the question again and amend your answer if necessary. This approach will allow you to secure a reasonable number of marks per section on questions that you are confident with (such as those that are shorter and easier to interpret) before spending time on more complicated questions.
- Be aware that you must read the whole screen of the question that you are on, otherwise you cannot move on to the next question or go back to any of the questions you have answered. There are both vertical and horizontal scroll bars.
- Before you start the test, you should be provided with a mini whiteboard, or as is the case in many test centres, a laminated piece of paper. Since the questions must be completed on a computer, there is no option to highlight or underline key points. In this case, the whiteboard or laminated paper provides a useful tool for jotting down any key points or components of calculations. Do not start the test without one, and if you feel it is necessary, ask for more! With the time pressures of the UCAT, even saving time by not having to rub away answers to previous questions can be incredibly valuable.
- It is worth keeping in mind that the precise scoring method is unknown as it is not information that the UCAT consortium shares. However, it is known that the score you obtain roughly corresponds to the number of questions you answer correctly. A maximum score of 900 is incredibly difficult to obtain, yet it is possible to score 900 and make some mistakes. A competitive score is generally viewed as anything above 700, as this is a difficult score to achieve and exceed.
- Finally, it is most important that you stay calm in the test. Prepare yourself, pace yourself and move on if you're struggling with

particular questions. It is inevitable that you will find some questions and some sections easier than others. In the same vein, perspective is important – the UCAT score is one aspect of a series of factors that will enable you to study medicine and is not the single most important part of your application.

Below is a summary of each subtest, with sample questions provided courtesy of Kaplan Test Prep.

Verbal Reasoning

The Verbal Reasoning test is designed to assess your ability to read and think carefully about information, using comprehension passages to get you to draw specific conclusions from the information presented. The test is based upon the verbal reasoning skills required of doctors to take on board often complex information, to analyse it and then to communicate in simple terms to patients and their families. There are 11 text passages which all have four questions to answer. Some questions will test your comprehension skills by asking you to answer 'true', 'false' or 'can't tell'. In general, if a similar statement can be found in the passage, it is true; if it opposes the information in the text, it is false; and if there is no direct reference to the statement in the passage, we can conclude that we can't tell from the information provided. The other type of question tests your critical response and will look for you to draw a conclusion. You will be presented with an incomplete statement or a question and four response options. You need to pick the most suitable response.

The verbal reasoning section is incredibly challenging, as it requires a rapid pace to get through lengthy passages of text and draw conclusions. In reality, you are unlikely to have much spare time on this section, so it is important to answer each question as you move through, even if it is a guess, rather than wasting time by moving backwards and forwards through questions.

Some candidates prefer to scan-read the passage before reading the questions, as this minimises the time spent reading the questions. Other candidates find this complicated, as it is difficult to remember all of the information in the passage. It may therefore be beneficial to scan-read the statement before looking for phrases relating to it in the passage. It is really important that you practise as many questions as possible, as this will allow you to identify particular strategies that work for you for each question type.

UCAT Verbal Reasoning Practice Questions

Subtest length: 44 questions (11 sets of 4 questions)
Subtest timing: 21 minutes (2 minutes per set)
Sample length: 4 questions
Sample timing: 2 minutes

In 1584, the rediscovery of the works of Tacitus led to the discovery of an old British heroic warrior, Boudicca. No mention is made of Boudicca, also known as Boadicea, in accounts of British history before the Renaissance, but she is referenced in three Roman works: Agricola *and* The Annals *by Tacitus and* The Rebellion of Boudicca *by Dio. Thus, since the time of Elizabeth I, another of England's great warrior queens, Boudicca has become a part of England's national history.*

Boudicca was the wife of Prasutagus, the head of the Iceni tribe in East England. In the year 43 CE when the Romans invaded England, Prasutagus was one of only two Celtic kings to retain some of his power, and the Romans gave him a grant. The Romans later redefined the grant as a loan, and, when Prasutagus died in 60 CE, he left half of his kingdom to Nero in payment, and the remainder to his daughters. When the Romans came to collect, they seized control of the kingdom, and attacked both Boudicca and her daughters.

Boudicca retaliated by attacking the Roman military's British operational base in Camulodunum, while most of the Roman army was away fighting in Wales. Boudicca's army drove out the Romans and burned Camulodunum to the ground. Boudicca and her army then attacked Londinium; Boudicca had the city burned to the ground and its entire population massacred. The ancient cities of Camulodunum and Londinium were later rebuilt and have since developed into Colchester and London, respectively.

Today, a bronze statue of Boudicca, commissioned during Victoria's reign and unveiled in 1905, stands alongside Westminster Bridge and the Houses of Parliament. The statue carries an inscription from William Cowper's 1782 poem Boadicea, an Ode: 'Regions Caesar never knew / Thy posterity shall sway.' Ironically, England's early anti-imperialist warrior became a primary cultural symbol for the British Empire, and today she stands over the city she once completely destroyed.

1. The British Empire expanded during Victoria's reign.

A. True B. False C. Can't tell

2. Following the Roman invasion, Boudicca's husband was allowed to keep some authority over his kingdom.

A. True B. False C. Can't tell

3. Roman forces in ancient Britain were headquartered in what is present-day London.

A. True B. False C. Can't tell

4. Some Roman historians took note of a foreign warrior queen.

A. True B. False C. Can't tell

Decision Making

This test assesses a candidate's ability to apply logic to reach a decision or conclusion, evaluate arguments and analyse statistical information.

A number of skills will be assessed in the decision making element of the UCAT, including:

- deductive reasoning
- evaluating arguments
- statistical reasoning
- figural reasoning.

These skills are assessed through a number of question types:

Logical puzzles

With these questions, you are required to make a deductive inference to arrive at a conclusion. It will involve solving a worded puzzle where some information is given, and the rest you are required to solve. When approaching these questions, you should:

- aim to identify the placement of known facts initially, so that they can be used as a reference for the placement of unknown facts
- eliminate any answers that you know cannot be true
- draw out the information using your whiteboard
- only do the working out that is required – if you do not need to complete the whole puzzle to get the answer, don't waste your time!

Syllogisms

Syllogisms are a form of reasoning where a conclusion is drawn based on a given premise: you are given a statement and asked to draw conclusions based on it. When answering these questions, you should:

- make sure that you have a thorough understanding of the premises given, reading them multiple times if required
- read the conclusions carefully and one by one, so that you can decide whether it is true or false after careful consideration
- avoid making assumptions
- pay attention to the use of qualifying terms.

These questions require a 'drag and drop' response. While it seems straightforward, you should make sure that you spend some time practising this using online practice versions of the test.

Interpreting information

With these questions, information will be presented – the form can vary considerably from passages of text to pie charts – and you must interpret it. You will be expected to draw conclusions based on this information. To increase your chances of getting these questions right, you should:

- try to ignore additional information that is given but is not required
- be prepared to use reasoning skills as opposed to prior knowledge
- where possible, round numbers to solve numerical problems as this will save time calculating
- try not to fall into the trap of basing your answers on the believability of a statement that is made.

Recognising assumptions

In these questions, you will be presented with a number of arguments and you are expected to choose the strongest one. To succeed in these questions, you should:

- ignore your prior beliefs as you must base your responses on the information presented to you
- remember that strong arguments will directly relate to the content in the questions, and this is what you should look out for
- remember assumptions will not be correct, so be careful not to select those as your answer.

Venn diagrams

You will be presented with a Venn diagram and you will be asked to draw conclusions from the information presented within it. You can improve your performance in these questions by:

- revisiting this area of maths and revise it thoroughly
- drawing your own Venn diagram to visualise the answer options.

Probabilistic reasoning

In these questions, you will be given some information containing statistical information and will be required to select the most appropriate response. You should:

- revisit the topic of probability and revise it thoroughly
- eliminate any obviously incorrect statements.

UCAT Decision Making Practice Questions

Subtest length: 29 questions (individual items, rather than sets)
Subtest timing: 31 minutes (1 minute per question)
Sample length: 3 questions
Sample timing: 3 minutes

1. *Vaccine K can prevent 88% of cases of Condition I, but cannot prevent 17% of cases of Condition II.*

Vaccine L cannot prevent 11% of cases of Condition I.

Vaccine L can prevent 86% of cases of Condition II.

Based on the success rates **only**, is Vaccine K more effective than Vaccine L at preventing the conditions?

A. Yes, because Vaccine K prevents more cases of both conditions.
B. Yes, because Vaccine K prevents more cases of Condition I than Vaccine L does.
C. No, because Vaccine L is more successful at preventing both conditions.
D. No, because Vaccine L is significantly more successful at preventing Condition II, but not Condition I.

2. Should train stations be allowed to charge for the use of the station toilets, which are an essential resource to all passengers who have already paid for a ticket?

Select the strongest argument from the statements below.

A. Yes, because the cost of cleaning and maintaining the toilets is considerable.
B. Yes, because most toilets are located in a part of the station that can be accessed by anyone, whether or not they have bought a ticket.
C. No, because passengers can use the toilets available on the trains.
D. No, because not everyone uses the toilets in train stations.

3. Some freshwater fish in the minnow family (Cyprinidae), such as the zebrafish, can regenerate their fins, heart or spinal cord following injury or amputation without any mutation or scarring thanks to fibroblast, a specialised protein that acts as a growth factor.

Place 'Yes' if the conclusion does follow. Place 'No' if the conclusion does not follow.

Minnows can regenerate after an injury without any scars.	
If a fish is a freshwater fish, it contains fibroblast.	
Some members of the family Cyprinidae are freshwater fish.	
Zebrafish can survive any injury by regenerating.	
A protein could allow certain minnows to replace an amputated fin.	

Quantitative Reasoning

The Quantitative Reasoning test is designed to see if you can solve problems using numerical skills. The test requires you to have good maths skills and knowledge of GCSE level maths. That is not the main point of this test, however; it is more a problem-solving exercise in terms of taking information and manipulating it with calculations and ratios.

As doctors are always using data, it is necessary to test this faculty. From drug calculations to medical research, applicants need to be able to show they have the ability to cope and can respond to different scenarios.

The data will be presented in a variety of ways, including tables, charts and graphs. Not all of the information provided will be immediately obvious, and it will require your close attention to detail to interpret them. Some data sets may not be presented visually at all, and you will be required to pick out the information from passages of text.

While there is some expectation of mathematical ability, you do not have to be exceptionally good at maths to perform well in the quantitative reasoning section. What is more important is being able to identify the appropriate information in the question and avoid making minor errors through carelessness, which is easily done in the time-pressured environment. In fact, some questions may not require you to do any calculations at all, but rather pick out information from visual data such as graphs and pie charts. Many of the calculations are relatively simple, and can be done by estimating.

A major drawback of the numerical reasoning component of the test is the on-screen calculator. Practising using an on-screen calculator in preparation is key for familiarising yourself with the test. While it only takes a few seconds longer than using an ordinary calculator, time is of the essence with this section, so any time that can be saved by carrying out calculations mentally will be incredibly valuable!

Sample questions are provided below. There are nine sets, each containing four questions, and you will have to choose between five answers. It is a practice-driven section and, as with maths, the more practice you do, the better.

It is worth committing a small proportion of your preparation time to reviewing your knowledge of some key mathematical skills and practising your mental maths so that you are more confident in your approach to more straightforward calculations.

- Being able to convert between percentages and fractions.
- Calculating the area of shapes, e.g. quadrilaterals, triangles and circles.
- Calculating the perimeter of shapes.
- Calculating the circumference of a circle.
- Calculating the volume of an object.
- Calculating percentages.
- Calculating percentage change.

UCAT Quantitative Reasoning Practice Questions

Subtest length: 36 questions (9 sets of 4 questions)
Subtest timing: 24 minutes (2 minutes per set)
Sample length: 4 questions
Sample timing: 2 minutes

The table indicates the total cost of renting different types of helicopter for a particular number of hours. Total cost equals the deposit plus the cost of renting per hour. Some information in the table is missing.

Type	Hours	Deposit	Hourly Rate	Total Cost
A	3	–	£500	£1,680
B	5	£240	£650	–
C	8	–	£4,895	£7,600
D	12	£5,675	£1,100	£13,875

1. Ian's total cost of renting a Type B helicopter was £4,790. For how many hours did he rent the helicopter?

A. 2
B. 3
C. 5
D. 7
E. 9

2. What is the ratio of the total cost of renting a Type A helicopter for 8 hours to the total cost of renting a Type C helicopter for 8 hours?

A. 10:19
B. 11:20
C. 3:5
D. 12:19
E. 8:11

3. The total cost of a Type D helicopter is discounted by a certain rate if rented for 24 hours. Jenni rents a Type D helicopter for 24 hours, with a total cost of £22,743. How much is the discount?

A. 16%
B. 18%
C. 20%
D. 22%
E. 24%

4. Type E helicopters have the same deposit as Type A helicopters. The cost per hour of a Type E helicopter is 25% more than for a Type A helicopter. What is the total cost of renting a Type E helicopter for 6 hours?

A. £2,430
B. £2,520
C. £3,930
D. £4,080
E. £4,200

Abstract Reasoning

Abstract Reasoning is designed to assess whether you can look at abstract shapes and then identify patterns, while ignoring the irrelevant material to avoid arriving at the wrong conclusion. What this test aims to do is test whether you are able to change your stance, be critical in your evaluations and create a hypothesis through inquiry.

Patients often give doctors numerous symptoms that doctors have to work through to work out what is relevant and what is not in order to arrive at a diagnosis. Doctors therefore have to use their judgement, as patients are not always accurate in the information they provide.

The patterns that you can be presented with will vary considerably, and some patterns will be far more complex than others. The ability to rapidly identify patterns comes easier to some people than others, but the key is to practise: the more patterns you see and become familiar with, the more readily you will be able to identify them. The abstract reasoning section is the fastest on the whole UCAT exam, so preparation is key!

In the UCAT test, you may see one of four items.

- **Type 1:** Two sets of shapes labelled 'Set A' and 'Set B'. From a test shape, you need to decide which set the shape belongs to, or neither.
- **Type 2:** From a series of shapes, you need to select the next shape in the series.
- **Type 3:** A statement will be given about a group of shapes and you then need to conclude which shape would complete the statement.
- **Type 4:** Two sets of shapes will be given to you labelled 'Set A' and 'Set B' and you need to decide from four options which belongs to Set A or Set B.

When approaching abstract reasoning questions, the most important aspect is to identify the pattern in each set. The easiest way of doing this is to pick two shapes – it is advisable to choose the most simplistic – and identify what is common about them. Each set will include shapes that are redundant and play no role in the pattern, so you must get used to ignoring these. For some shapes, there will be one common feature, whereas others may have multiple. These can be to do with the number, size, orientation, positioning and colour of the shapes, as well as the shapes themselves.

UCAT Abstract Reasoning Practice Questions

Subtest length: 55 questions (11 sets of 5 questions)
Subtest timing: 13 minutes (1 minute per set)
Sample length: 5 questions
Sample timing: 1 minute

Set A ***Set B***

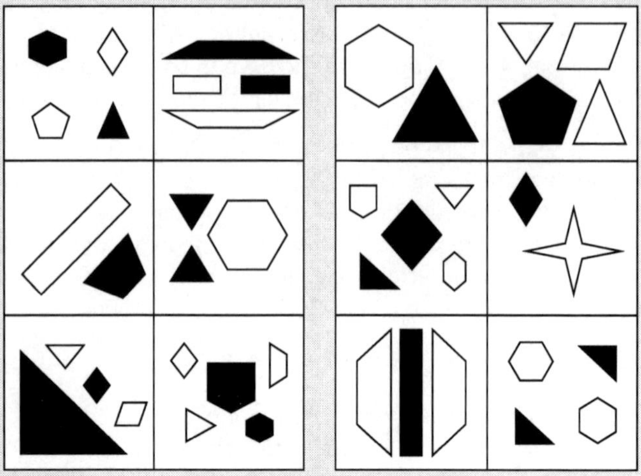

Test Shapes

1 2 3 4 5

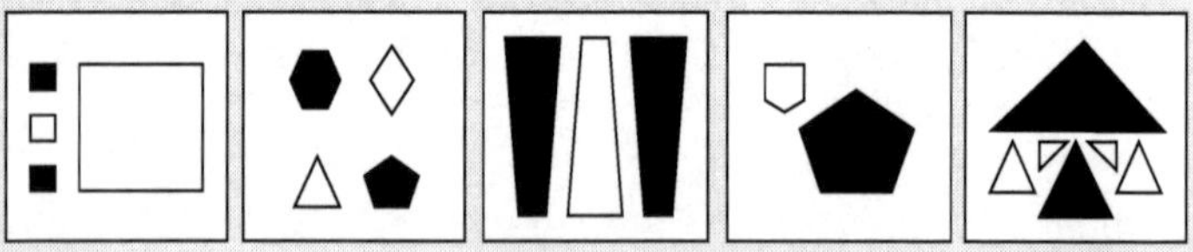

1	2	3	4	5
o A. Set A	o A. Set A	o A. Set A	o A. Set A	o A. Set A
o B. Set B	o B. Set B	o B. Set B	o B. Set B	o B. Set B
o C. Neither	o C. Neither	o C. Neither	o C. Neither	o C. Neither

Situational Judgement

The Situational Judgement Test is designed to measure how you deal with real-world situations and whether you can identify critical factors and apply appropriate behaviour in the handling of them. What it is ultimately measuring is the level of integrity and perspective you will bring to the profession and whether you are able to work in a multi-disciplinary team.

The score of the Situational Judgement Test is recorded as a 'band', with band 1 representing the highest score and band 4 representing the lowest. These scores are not included in the UCAT average score but are recorded independently and, as such, are typically used separately by medical schools.

You will be presented with 22 different scenarios and each one will have different actions that you could take, with varying considerations. Typically, these considerations will be in line with maintaining a consistently high level of professionalism, having an understanding of medical ethics and recognising the importance of patient safety. There is no expectation that you will have the procedural knowledge to answer these, but it is worth remembering a few key points.

- Under no circumstances should a doctor, or any other medical professional, carry out any action that may affect the confidence of patients in the profession.
- Problems must be addressed as quickly as possible to reassure the patient.
- Where possible, solutions must be identified and put into place efficiently.

The Situational Judgement Test is often viewed as the easiest section, but it should not be underestimated. One reason is that this is the final section of the examination, and you are likely to be fatigued by this point and therefore more likely to make mistakes. In addition, it is a busy section with a large quantity of scenarios in a short period of time. Finally, it may be that each of the possible answers seems plausible, so it is difficult to identify which one is correct.

In the first set of questions, you have to determine the 'appropriateness' of the options in the given scenario. You will be given the following four options to give as your response.

1. **A very appropriate thing to do:** you should give this answer if it addresses at least one aspect of the scenario; it does not have to be all aspects.
2. **Appropriate, but not ideal:** you should give this answer if it was not an ideal solution, though it could be done, despite not being best practice.
3. **Inappropriate, but not awful:** you should give this answer if it should not be done, though it would not be considered terrible.
4. **A very inappropriate thing to do:** you should give this answer if you should definitely not do this.

In giving a response (i.e. 1–4), always remember that it might not be the only course of action and you should not consider it as such.

In the second set, you need to rate the 'importance' of a number of choices regarding a given scenario. You will be given the following four options to give as your response.

1. **Very important:** you would give this answer if this is vital to take into account.
2. **Important:** you would give this answer if it was important but not vital to take into account.
3. **Of minor importance:** you would give this answer if you should take it into account but it would not matter if it was not considered.
4. **Not important at all:** you would give this answer if you should definitely not be taking this information into account.

When approaching these questions, you should consider:

- the appropriateness or importance of the action
- whether the action actually addresses the problem at hand
- whether there are any possible unintended consequences associated with the action.

In addition to the above, the Situational Judgement section has recently introduced a number of scenarios that are answered through a 'drag-and-drop' format: each question has multiple components and you must drag the correct answer and drop it into each component.

UCAT Situational Judgement Practice Questions

Subtest length: 20 scenarios, 2 to 5 questions each (69 questions total)
Subtest timing: 26 minutes (20–30 seconds per scenario, then 10–15 seconds per question)
Sample length: 4 questions
Sample timing: 1 minute

A medical student, Emmet, is completing a patient history as part of his placement at a GP surgery. The patient has previously been treated for emphysema and has difficulty breathing, but he has continued to smoke. The patient mentions that the doctor 'keeps telling me to quit' but insists that he enjoys cigarettes, they help him to relax, and 'you're not taking away my one pleasure in life'. Emmet has experience as a volunteer on a stop smoking campaign, so he feels qualified to engage with the patient on this issue.

How **appropriate** are each of the following responses by Emmet in this situation?

1. Discuss other relaxing activities, such as reading, music or sport, that the patient might enjoy.

A. A very appropriate thing to do
B. Appropriate, but not ideal
C. Inappropriate, but not awful
D. A very inappropriate thing to do

2. Tell the patient that he risks shortening his life, with reduced quality of life, if he keeps smoking.

A. A very appropriate thing to do

B. Appropriate, but not ideal

C. Inappropriate, but not awful

D. A very inappropriate thing to do

3. Remind the patient that the doctors know best and he would do well to follow their advice.

A. A very appropriate thing to do

B. Appropriate, but not ideal

C. Inappropriate, but not awful

D. A very inappropriate thing to do

Verbal Reasoning Practice Questions - Answers

1. (C)
2. (A)
3. (B)
4. (A)

Decision Making Practice Questions - Answers

1. (C)
2. (B)
3. NO; NO; YES; NO; YES

Quantitative Reasoning Practice Questions - Answers

1. (D)
2. (B)
3. (A)
4. (C)

Abstract Reasoning Practice Questions - Answers

1. (A)
2. (C)
3. (C)
4. (A)
5. (B)

Situational Judgement Practice Questions - Answers

1. (A)
2. (B)
3. (D)

All practice questions provided by Kaplan Test Prep, a leading provider of preparation for the UCAT and BMAT. See www.kaptest.com/ucat to learn more about preparing with Kaplan Test Prep.

How do universities use the UCAT?

The utilisation of UCAT scores varies considerably between the different medical schools, and the guidance tends to change slightly each year. It is therefore crucial that the information provided here is utilised alongside that on the websites of the medical schools, as well as the information provided by the UCAT consortium.

If you have underperformed in the UCAT, obtaining an average score of less than the average, which is typically around 630, it is not the end of the road for your medicine application. You should focus on universities that put more weighting in the selection process on other aspects of your application, and so do not focus on the UCAT score quite as much. For example, Cardiff University ranks applicants based on their academic performance, using the UCAT score only in borderline cases.

Below are some examples of the ways in which the UCAT has been used by medical schools.

University of Birmingham

The University of Birmingham does not use a cut-off score, but instead uses the overall UCAT score from the four subtests to rank applicants. They divide UCAT scores into deciles based on the applicant pool, then allocate their own score to each of the deciles.

For guidance, the decile boundaries in 2020–21 are outlined in Table 5 (below). It is worth noting that the scores will change depending on the applicants each year, though this provides a useful framework.

Table 5 Guidance on UCAT scoring

Total UCAT score	Decile	Converted score
2860 and above	10th	4.000
2740–2850	9th	3.556
2650–2730	8th	3.111
2580–2640	7th	2.667
2510–2570	6th	2.222

2440–2500	5th	1.778
2370–2430	4th	1.333
2280–2360	3rd	0.889
2160–2270	2nd	0.444
2150 and below	1st	0.000

University of Bristol

All applicants are required to take the UCAT exam for consideration by the University of Bristol. They make use of the total UCAT score from each of the four subtests in order to select for interview. Though the threshold score used for the interview cut-off changes each year, for 2023 entry it was 2910 for home applicants and 2960 for overseas applicants.

University of East Anglia

All applicants must sit the UCAT in the year that they apply to the University of East Anglia. They do not use a cut-off score, but outline that a high score would be advantageous, though a low score would not disqualify an applicant either. As with the other universities discussed above, it is the overall UCAT score from the four subtests that is used to rank applicants for selection for interview. It is then used again alongside interview scores to determine who should be made an offer. It is important to note that the Situational Judgement component of the UCAT is combined with the interview score.

The Situational Judgement Test

Although most students focus on the average UCAT score consideration of medical schools, many schools now also look at performance on the SJT.

Several universities do not consider performance on the SJT at all. At the time of writing, these include:

- Aston University
- University of Bristol
- University of Plymouth
- Queen's University Belfast (except to help with borderline applicants in 2023 and may be used for 2024 entry)
- University of Southampton
- St George's, University of London.

Medical schools that do use the SJT tend to only do so in the case of obtaining a Band 4, which results in rejection. These universities include:

- University of Aberdeen
- Anglia Ruskin University
- Brunel University

- Edge Hill University
- University of Edinburgh
- Hull York Medical School
- Keele University
- University of Leicester
- University of Lincoln
- University of Liverpool (with the exception of international applicants)
- University of Manchester
- Newcastle University
- University of Nottingham
- University of Sunderland.

A number of universities, including Cardiff University and the University of Exeter, do not provide any formal guidance on how the SJT is used. While it is most likely to be the case that it is not used, it is worth approaching these universities with caution in the case of a poor SJT score.

As well as being used to make outright decisions, performance in the SJT can also influence whether or not you are invited to interview. The following universities demonstrate a specific scoring mechanism whereby the SJT score contributes:

- University of Edinburgh
- Hull York Medical School
- King's College, London
- University of Lincoln
- University of Nottingham.

Similarly, the SJT can also influence the interview process directly. In some cases, a high SJT score would place you at an advantage at the interview stage, even if it did not contribute to getting you the interview in the first place. Medical schools that will scrutinise applicants with a low SJT score more heavily at interview include:

- University of Birmingham
- University of East Anglia
- Hull York Medical School
- Queen Mary University of London
- University of Sheffield
- University of St Andrews.

It is important to note that this information is accurate at the time of writing, but you should always check with each individual university to ensure that their stance regarding the importance of the SJT has not changed.

UCAT fees

- Test taken in the UK: £70
- Test taken outside the UK: £115

This information is accurate at the time of writing.

UCAT SJTace

The Situational Judgement Test for Admission to Clinical Education was taken up for 2018/19 by the universities of Dundee and St Andrews for their Scottish Graduate Entry Medical (ScotGEM) programme. It is designed to select the candidates who they deem to have the right professional behaviour necessary to be successful in the medical profession. It is identical to the Situational Judgement Test in the standard UCAT test.

BMAT (BioMedical Admissions Test)

The BMAT is a test to ensure effective selection of well-qualified students. This is a written test and is deemed a productive indicator of a student's likely result in their first year of undergraduate study.

Up until October 2023, Cambridge Assessment Admissions Testing ran the BMAT, an alternative entrance exam, which was used by six UK universities. October 2023 marked the final test date for the BMAT as it stands, with no alternative test provider stepping in to replace it at the time of writing. It is still possible that a different provider will produce the test, or that the universities that have used it up until this point will utilise an alternative means of assessing students, such as the UCAT.

The UK medical schools that used the BMAT were:

- Brighton and Sussex Medical School
- Imperial College London
- Lancaster University
- University College London
- University of Cambridge
- University of Oxford.

At the time of writing, some of these universities have not outlined what they will use in place of the BMAT. However, the University of Leeds has already switched to the UCAT for 2024 entry, and University College London has indicated that it too will switch to the UCAT for 2025 entry. Imperial College London is currently reviewing its entry criteria for 2025 and will publish this in time for the 2024 cycle, though its decision had not been made at the time of writing.

5 | The personal statement

One of the most important parts of your application is your personal statement, as this is your chance to show the university selectors three very important themes. These are:

- why you want to be a doctor
- what you have done to investigate the profession
- whether you are the right sort of person for their medical school (i.e. the personal qualities that make you an outstanding candidate).

The personal statement is your opportunity to demonstrate to the admissions tutors not only that you have researched medicine thoroughly, but that you also have the right personal qualities to succeed as a doctor, you are fully committed to studying medicine and have the right motivation and personal qualities to do so successfully. A typical personal statement takes time and effort to get right; don't expect perfection after one draft.

When it comes to distinguishing between highly qualified candidates, one of the most important factors that is considered is the personal statement. If this is badly worded, littered with errors or lacking detail about the attributes and experiences of the candidate, it will stand a chance of being rejected without being taken further. Ultimately, this means that the more thought that you give to your UCAS application and personal statement, the better they will be and the greater your chance of being asked to come in for an interview and being made a conditional offer.

The personal statement is expected to be replaced with a set of questions in the future (but no earlier than the 2024/25 application cycle for 2026 entry). At the time of writing, UCAS has indicated that these are likely to cover:

- motivation for the course and why you want to study it
- preparedness for the course and how your learning to date has set you up for success
- preparation through other experiences, such as work or voluntary experience or extracurricular activities
- extenuating circumstances
- preparedness for study and what you have done to prepare yourself for life as an undergraduate student
- preferred learning style and how your chosen course is suitable.

For the most part, these questions broadly cover the areas that are covered in the personal statement in its current format, but with guided structure.

Sections of the personal statement

Why medicine?

Your personal statement must, fundamentally, convince admissions tutors of your interest in following a career in medicine.

A high proportion of UCAS applications contain a sentence like 'From an early age I have wanted to be a doctor because it is the only career that combines my love of science with the chance to work with people.' Not only do admissions tutors get bored with reading this, it doesn't necessarily highlight your desire to study medicine: there are many careers that combine science and people, including teaching, pharmacy, physiotherapy and nursing.

However, the basic ideas behind this sentence may well apply to you. If so, you need to personalise it. You could mention an incident that first got you interested in medicine – a visit to your own doctor, a conversation with a family friend, or a lecture at school, for instance. You could write about your interest in human biology or a biology project that you undertook when you were younger to illustrate your interest in science, and you could give examples of how you like to work with others. The important thing is to back up your initial interest with your efforts to investigate the career.

It is a common misconception that you need to begin your personal statement with an inspirational quotation or grand statement; again, admissions tutors get bored of students trying to squeeze in lines from books, poems or films that have no real meaning to the applicant. What an admissions tutor would rather see is a statement of the genuine reasons that you want to study medicine, written in clear, uncomplicated English.

Another common pitfall in the first paragraph is taking up valuable space with an explanation about what the subject is about or what the profession entails. For example: 'Medicine is a highly regarded profession that involves the diagnosis, treatment and prevention of disease.' Remember that the people reading your statement know exactly what the profession is about and so do not need to be lectured on it! Instead, you need to take the time to explain about your own interest in the profession and why you feel compelled to follow this career path.

Finally, don't be afraid to lean on your work experience placements or voluntary work here. Often, those initial sparks of interest in a career in medicine are underpinned by what you observed when shadowing a doctor in A&E, or when you were playing board games with elderly patients in a care home. This section of the personal statement should be sizeable, so it is a good idea to link your motivation to study medicine in with your experiences of healthcare. These experiences will also form a significant proportion of your personal statement.

Work experience and voluntary work

This section is important to demonstrate that you gained something from your work experience and voluntary placements, and that they have given you an insight into the profession. Start by talking about your medicine-specific experiences. You should give an indication of the length of time you spent at each placement and the impressions you gained. You could comment on what aspects of medicine attract you, or on what you found interesting or something that you hadn't expected, but remember that this is not a shopping list. You are not simply reeling off experience after experience; you are expected to provide deeper reflection about what you have seen. Beyond this, you should also mention any other work experience or voluntary work you have had in a caring or clinical role and what you learned from it. Although you may not think of these sorts of experiences as being relevant, they can often demonstrate to an admissions tutor good interpersonal skills or commitment and dedication, all of which are relevant to medicine.

Here is a sample description of a student's work experience that would probably not impress the admissions team.

> *'I spent three days at my local GP surgery. I saw a patient have their blood pressure taken. It was very interesting.'*

In contrast, the example below would be much more convincing because it is clear that the student was interested in what was happening.

> *'During a two-week placement at my local GP surgery, I shadowed two GPs and a clinical nurse. As well as being able to observe how the doctors and nurses interacted with anxious and unwell patients, I was able to witness a number of medical interventions, including blood samples being taken, blood pressure being measured and a referral recommendation to a specialist doctor following a patient's complaints of back pain. What I found particularly interesting was the fact that, although both doctors had very different personalities, they both related well to the patients, who seemed to find them very reassuring. A number of things surprised me; in particular, how varying a doctor's day can be.'*

Spelling mistakes, grammatical errors and unclear personal statements will create an unfavourable impression on the selectors. In order to ensure that this does not happen, follow these tips.

It will be far easier to write this section of your personal statement if you kept notes in a reflective journal during your work experience as discussed previously. Look back over what you wrote and use your thoughts and experiences as a stimulus for this section. With luck, the admissions tutors may pick up on these experiences at interview and ask you to expand on some of your comments.

Following this, you should discuss the experiences you have had whilst undertaking any voluntary work. Any type of voluntary placement is a useful addition to your statement, but ongoing work in a care-based or clinical setting really boosts your profile. Opportunities often exist in care homes, children's hospices and hospitals and it is worth trying to contribute regularly over a long period of time rather than carrying it out for just a week or two. This type of experience can help you get an insight into patient care and the communication side of the profession and gives a really good opportunity to discuss how your interpersonal skills have developed whilst working with people. As with any medical work experience, you should make a note of any key experiences that you have and what they have taught you, as this can then be commented on in your personal statement.

Your academic interests

It is important for your personal statement to contain information about your academic interests and how they have furthered your desire to study medicine. This may be related to some topics or practical skills that have been of particular interest to you over the course of your A level studies, or to an interesting article you have read in a newspaper or journal, or to something engaging you heard in a lecture. Whatever it is, it will help to demonstrate your desire to pursue the course, as long as you make it relevant to medicine and put in sufficient detail. In so many personal statements this section struggles to get beyond 'I enjoyed learning about the human body' and 'I enjoy using different apparatus in practical work'; however, this is too generic to be meaningful. Keeping a journal over a long period of time of any wider reading that is relevant to medicine will help this section to genuinely reflect what your interests are rather than being based on what you have panic-read the week before submitting your application.

Evidence of developing skills and personal qualities

The person reading your UCAS application has to decide two things: whether you have the right skills and personal qualities to become a successful doctor, and whether you will be able to cope with and contribute to medical school life. To be a successful medic, you need (among other things!) to:

- successfully pass your undergraduate studies
- have good interpersonal skills and get on with a wide range of people
- be able to work under pressure and cope with stress
- have well-developed manual skills.

How, then, does the person reading your personal statement know whether you have the qualities they are looking for? What you must remember is that the admissions tutor doesn't know you, so you have to give lots of evidence of how you have demonstrated and developed these qualities. Some of the things they may be looking for are:

- skill development during work experience/voluntary work
- positions of responsibility
- work in the local community
- an ability to get on with people
- participation in activities involving manual dexterity
- participation in team events
- involvement in school plays or concerts.

Some examples of aspects that you might want to include in your application are detailed below.

Have you demonstrated a range of interests?

Medical schools like to see applicants who have done more with their life than work for their A levels and watch TV. While the teacher writing your reference will probably refer to your outstanding academic achievements, you also need to say something about your achievements in your personal statement. Admissions tutors like to read about achievements in sport and other outdoor activities, such as the Duke of Edinburgh's Award Scheme. Equally useful activities include Young Enterprise, charity work, public speaking, part-time jobs, art, music and drama.

Bear in mind that admissions tutors will be asking themselves: 'Would this person be an asset to the medical school?' Put in enough detail and try to make it interesting to read. An important point to note though is that extra-curricular information must not take up more than about 25% of your personal statement, as the primary focus is on why you want to get in to medicine.

The key is to ensure that you are always relating your personal qualities and extra-curricular activities to your application, in order to show evidence of the attributes and skills needed to become a doctor. It needs to be relevant to the medical application, to demonstrate to admission tutors that you are the right sort of person for the university.

Here is an example of a good paragraph on interests for the personal statement section:

> *'I very much enjoy tennis and play in the school team and for Hampshire at under-18 level. This summer a local sports shop has sponsored me to attend a tennis camp in California. I worked at*

the Wimbledon championships in 2016. Doing so has placed the emphasis of team work and personal reliance on me. I have been playing the piano since the age of eight and took my Grade 7 exam recently, which I think demonstrates manual dexterity. At school, I play in the orchestra and in a very informal jazz band. Last year I started learning the trombone but I would not like anyone except my teacher to hear me playing! Music is a perfect way to relax; at the same time, it got me thinking about the link between music and medicine. The discipline and dedication of years of practice required in both is similar – not to mention the manual dexterity integral in each – but more so, looking into it, I have become fascinated by the link between the two, both from a therapeutic perspective – music therapy for example being a new technique designed to interact with patients – and a relaxation standpoint; anything from the music in a doctor's waiting room to the music playing in an operating room to calm the surgeon and help them focus. I like dancing and social events but my main form of relaxation is gardening. I have started a small business helping my neighbours to improve their gardens – which also brings in some extra money.'

And here's how not to do it:

'I play tennis in competitions and the piano and trombone. I like gardening.'

But what if you aren't musical, can't play tennis and find geraniums boring? It depends when you are reading this. Anyone with enough drive to become a doctor can probably rustle up an interest or two in six months. If you haven't even got that long, then it would be sensible to devote most of your personal statement to your interest in medicine.

Have you contributed to school activities?

This is largely covered by the section on interests, but it is worth noting that the selector is looking for someone who will contribute to the communal life of the medical school. If you have been involved in organising things in your school, include the details. Don't forget to say that you ran the school's fundraising barbecue or that you organised guest speakers for the college medical society. Conversely, medical schools are less interested in applicants whose activities are exclusively solitary or cannot take place in the medical school environment.

The admissions tutors will be aware that some schools offer more to their students in the way of activities and responsibilities than others. However, even if there are very few opportunities made available to you through your school, you must still find ways to gain experience and develop your skills. You don't have to have been captain of the rugby team or gone on a three-month expedition to Borneo to be considered, but you do need to be able to demonstrate that you have made efforts to participate in a range of worthwhile activities.

Have you any achievements or leadership experience to your credit?

Admissions tutors are particularly attracted by excellence in any sphere. Have you competed in any activity at a high level or received a prize or other recognition for your achievements? Have you organised and led any events or team games? Were you elected as class representative to the school council? If so, make sure that you include it in your statement.

WARNING!

- Don't write anything that isn't true.
- Don't write anything you can't talk about at the interview.
- Avoid over-complicated, over-formal styles of writing. Read your personal statement out loud; if it doesn't sound like you speaking, rewrite it.

TIP!

Keep a copy of your personal statement so that you can look at it when you prepare for the interview.

Things to avoid

Writing your personal statement can be a difficult and long-winded process. There are some things easy to avoid that will ensure that you make a good impression with your application.

1. Not enough words.
   You must ensure that the personal statement is as close to the 4,000 character limit as possible. Anything significantly below the character count will make a negative impression on the admissions tutors.
2. A lack of detail or reflection.
   It is crucial that you do not simply list your experiences, but carefully reflect on them to ensure that the admissions tutors can see that you have gained a lot from them. When discussing work experience, go into detail about what you witnessed and reflect on what you learned. When giving details of what you are studying, be specific about topics you have enjoyed. This will give the admissions tutor a much greater insight into who you are and the skills you possess.
3. Not being very personal.
   Make sure your personal statement has evidence and experiences to show an admissions tutor who you really are and what you are genuinely interested in.

4. **Negativity.**
   Unfortunately, many personal statements contain negative points about things that an applicant hasn't enjoyed studying or things they might not like about the career. These are sometimes included due to a misguided need to be brutally honest, but this really is not necessary. The overall tone should be optimistic and positive throughout.
5. **Lecturing about medicine.**
   Statements that list facts about medicine or what doctors do can often waste space. Remember that the people reading your statement will know all of this. Use the space instead to illustrate from your own experiences that you possess the qualities and skills that doctors need.
6. **Discussing money and potential earnings.**
   Although most medicine applicants will have thought about how much money they will be making at some point, it is not something that needs to be highlighted in your personal statement. Your reasons for studying medicine need to run much deeper than this if you are going to get into medical school.
7. **The use of overused, repeated stock phrases.**
   Commonly used statements can make an admissions tutor question whether your statement is an accurate picture of who you are. If you genuinely want to express a generic idea, think of how you could expand on it in your own words to make it more meaningful.
8. **Losing the focus on medicine.**
   If the only place that really comes alive in your personal statement is when you are discussing how much you enjoy studying English Literature, then you are misusing the space that you have available. Transfer that enthusiasm to elements of your personal statement that the admissions tutors will want to see.
9. **Overusing the thesaurus.**
   Beware of overusing a thesaurus. Obviously, you want your English to be as good as possible, but make sure that what you have written makes sense and sounds like you.
10. **Use of Artificial Intelligence (AI).**
    When completing your UCAS application, you now have to declare that the personal statement is your own work, which includes not using AI software. The use of platforms such as ChatGPT could be deemed as cheating by universities and could impact whether your application is considered.

Four sample statements can be found on the following pages. The examples demonstrate clarity and focus, and what comes through the most is the enthusiasm that the candidates have for medicine. These attributes will give an applicant an excellent chance of being called in for an interview and/or just being given an offer.

Personal statement: Example 1 (character count: 3,981)

My motivation to pursue a career in medicine has developed from a desire to combine my scientific curiosity with the opportunity to enhance a person's quality of life. It is a privilege to undertake this career, and requires dedication, diligence and compassion. I have broadened my understanding of this exciting and dynamic profession through work experience and volunteering.

Spending time in an inner city General Practice, I witnessed the importance of a trusting doctor–patient relationship in a baby clinic. I observed the high prevalence of poor health outcomes in young mothers presenting with conditions such as diabetes and obesity. It was eye-opening to see the positive approach deployed by the GP, with optimism that she could encourage positive change in her patients. Another consultation, this time between the relatives of a dying patient and the GP, highlighted the proficient communication skills and empathy required to support families in distressing times. My experience in primary care made me appreciate the truly multidisciplinary nature of medicine. I observed a physiotherapist who led the assessment of patients with musculoskeletal complaints, bringing a complementary approach to the team; I appreciate that doctors can only work effectively as part of a unit with other allied health professionals, all aiming for the best outcomes.

Doctors must be compassionate, caring and have a sense of social responsibility. I experienced these qualities while volunteering at Chandos Primary School, where I mentored children with their reading skills. Forming connections with pupils was a fulfilling chance to practise my communication skills, while recognising the challenges facing children in our inner cities. Driven by my sense of community, I volunteered at a local food bank, where I organised and distributed groceries to those in need. These experiences have developed my sense of empathy and helped me become a more compassionate person.

I undertook work experience at Russells Hall Hospital, shadowing surgeons performing a keyhole knee operation. This experience showed me how modern medicine can lead to a profound improvement in quality of life. Within the operating theatre, I witnessed the seamless cooperation between the anaesthetist, the orthopaedic surgeon and nursing staff working towards a common goal. I also experienced this skill of coordinated teamwork when I played for the Warwickshire County Cricket Birmingham District team for five years and as a member of my school hockey team. Playing in these squads has tested my strength as a team member, and adapting to act as a captain has encouraged my own leadership skills.

There is a research aspect to medicine that interdigitates with clinical responsibilities. Eager to learn more about this, I organised work experience at the Angiogenesis Research Laboratory at Aston University. I was grateful to be accepted on a summer project investigating the use of microneedles as a method of drug delivery. This has led me to further research the benefit of this technology in improving diabetes care. I have gained insight into the academic research environment and its vital role in improving patient care.

Initiative and commitment are key attributes of a successful doctor. Continuing my passion for cricket, I successfully completed the ECB Support Coaching qualification and obtained paid employment as a coach to 7–11-year-olds at Harborne Cricket Club. This role has enhanced my sense of responsibility: keeping the children in a safe environment and making each session as interactive as possible. I have learnt to make appropriate decisions in a short time frame, which is a relevant attribute of clinical decision making.

Medicine is a challenging yet fulfilling career choice. I recognise that being a doctor requires resilience and a lifetime of sincere commitment. I believe my journey so far has shown I possess the qualities necessary to prosper in this ever-advancing field.

Personal statement: Example 2 (character count: 3,923)

My motivation to study medicine stemmed from my interest in its evolving nature, which I saw first-hand when shadowing a physiotherapist. I noticed this through the use of modern technology, where I observed the use of video games to create a more interactive experience for patients. I recognised that patients are more likely to view the outlook of their treatment more positively if they are enjoying it.

While completing work experience in a hospital, I noted the realities of healthcare work as I observed a patient's inability to communicate due to a stroke bringing them to tears. I was inspired by the doctor's determination to aid the patient, through non-verbal communication and techniques such as the use of close-ended questions. Using calming words and being understanding made the patient relax, which demonstrated the impact a doctor has on a patient's emotions. This experience taught me that it's the responsibility of the doctor to support a patient through difficult times by effective communication and resilience, despite any barriers. This builds trust, which reinforces patient-centred care.

Some patients in the UK can experience anxiety about healthcare situations due to language barriers. I have been responsible for translating for members of my family for many years. A specific case was when a family member had to pick up medicine from the GP and their language barrier prevented them from expressing their needs. Showing patience and understanding allowed us to communicate successfully, which I also noted during my work experience. I also used compassion to understand the struggles of having a verbal barrier, which is relevant when making sure patients have informed consent for procedures; this highlighted the importance of empathy to work in partnership with patients.

While studying Biology at A level, I was fascinated by the impact of diabetes and ways of managing life with diabetes. This led to me volunteering at a workshop to help those with diabetes to keep fit, where my passion further developed. It also reinforced the value of care when interacting with others. Demonstrating compassion meant that I could improve someone's day and cultivate good working relationships.

Teamwork is vital in medicine, as maintaining relationships is important when handing over roles in the MDT and ensures effective patient management. I saw teamwork and good communication in action when a patient's oxygen saturation was falling – the team considered the outcomes and worked together to prevent the condition from worsening. Similarly, when playing netball, there were times where we would communicate our favoured positions and occasionally compromise; in these situations, I vocalised my opinion, while listening to my teammates. This enabled us to be more productive, meaning that establishing a level of communication between the team meant we all felt satisfied.

To further my insight into the profession, I set up a conversation with a consultant, where I realised the significance of reflection and that to be a skilled doctor it is essential to be adaptive. Since then, I have strived to do this in many aspects of my life. Volunteering at a charity shop has helped build my confidence. My communication skills have vastly improved through the experiences with customers, but more so through my collaboration with the staff where I was able to meet and work with new people.

A career in medicine grants me the opportunity to work in a dynamic environment, which I feel well suited to. After gaining an insight into medicine, I recognise that being a doctor comes with a great responsibility and challenges, which is why resilience is essential. I am also aware of the importance of reflection, particularly in a constantly changing profession. Therefore, I look to apply these skills in the interest of making myself a successful future doctor.

Personal statement: Example 3 (character count: 3,812)

The psychological and social aspects of pain can play a greater part than the biological, highlighting the uniqueness of every patient's personal story. In my EPQ on pain, I learnt that a holistic approach is so important in medicine. This varied challenge and thrill of diagnostic reasoning, with countless treatment approaches, is what motivated me to pursue a career in the complex field of medicine. I then began to meticulously explore medicine through work experience and conversations with doctors and medical students.

Empathy is an essential skill in medicine, as it builds trust within the doctor–patient relationship, and I witnessed this as a volunteer in a care home. A carer was talking with a distressed elderly patient, and I noticed she used supportive language and reassured the patient. She mirrored the patient's tone and facial expressions to show understanding. I developed my own empathy skills through volunteering as a patient advocate for COVID vaccinations, where I spent extra time talking to anxious patients. I used a calm tone and open body language, which enabled them to feel at ease.

During my six-month virtual work experience with Medic Mentor, I shadowed a doctor in the ICU and recognised the importance of communication. When assessing a critically ill patient, the doctor used active listening and thoroughly explained the pros and cons of treatments in a non-biased way, enabling the patient to make an informed decision. While working at a children's holiday club, I furthered my communication skills by adapting to speaking with teachers, parents, and children. I enhanced my confidence in communication by gaining a distinction in my grade 8 LAMDA and as a maths mentor and Biology Scholar, where I simplified information into understandable chunks and used visual diagrams to explain concepts.

During my virtual work experience, I appreciated how good communication allowed the MDT to work cohesively, with everyone understanding their role and importance. The senior registrar effectively took the lead and delegated tasks, to ensure rapid treatment and patient safety. During my Gold DofE expedition, one of my team members fell ill, so I took responsibility to redistribute the roles, and get help swiftly.

As the first pastoral mentor in my school, I led a team of younger pupils, where we worked together to improve mental well-being through the teaching of the Peer Education Programme.

A week of virtual work experience at Birmingham Children's Hospital allowed me to understand the process of preparation and aftercare for surgery. This motivated me to complete an Open University MOOC on pain and aspirin. Following this, I attended a Cambridge University Masterclass on pain, which inspired me to undertake an EPQ on this topic. Through interviews with patients, I gained a greater awareness and empathy for those living with chronic pain.

I enjoy learning Arabic, I am working towards grade 5 violin and a black belt in karate. These activities have enabled me to appreciate different cultures while gaining physical and mental strength. This is important, as I learnt from *When Breath Becomes Air* by Kalanithi, because medicine involves dealing with uncertainty and will be emotionally and physically exhausting. I experienced this uncertainty first-hand when I missed my place for medicine due to achieving a B in Chemistry A level. After reflecting on the result, I decided to take a gap year to resit the A level and further my experience and skills through working in a GP Practice and with St John's Ambulance.

Despite facing this rejection, my enthusiasm to overcome the challenges of a career in medicine has only increased. The reward of life-long learning and compassion, combined with the honour of the profession, has made me even more determined to study medicine.

Personal statement: Example 4 (character count: 3,960)

My path into applying for medicine has been slightly unusual. I discovered that I wanted to study medicine while in my first year of an English Literature and French degree; I was enjoying my studies, but felt that something was missing. While working as a Notes Summariser at a GP practice, I found myself fascinated by the stories that patient records held and the impact of medical care on an individual's life. I wondered how it would feel to be involved in offering that care, and realised something missing from my future plans was the meaning that my life could offer to others. I found myself wanting to be in the position of the doctor, so that I could learn more about the world of medicine and help people similar to the individuals I was reading about. I decided, having successfully completed my first year at university, to leave and focus on my ambition of reading medicine, by studying A level Biology and Chemistry. This increased my desire to develop an understanding of medicine's scientific basis, while allowing me to improve my independent study skills which I had developed at university.

As I had already experienced Primary Care, I wanted to understand more about hospital medicine, and so arranged some work experience where I was given the opportunity to shadow a range of medical professionals. I was struck by the teamwork involved, with many different roles working together for the patient to make a successful healthcare service. I found shadowing in oncology thought-provoking, and I felt that the holistic nature of care was particularly important. In cardiology, I witnessed an encounter between a Registrar and an unhappy patient who wanted to go home, and noticed how by allowing them to express how they were feeling, comforting them, and then explaining clearly why they needed to remain in hospital, the situation was successfully resolved. I was able to observe a complicated operation to remove a tumour from the rectum of a patient, which highlighted the technical skill and scientific knowledge required. This was reinforced when I observed a stent being inserted into an artery to prevent a heart attack. It was such a quick operation, but talking to the surgeon afterwards, his comment that it could also be very quick to kill someone through the operation and the responsibility associated with that, has stayed with me.

Working as a Domiciliary Care Worker has given me the skills to manage the care of individuals on my own, and shown me the importance of companionship to those who are elderly or frail. Looking after people with dementia has taught me how to remain patient and clear when communicating.

My neighbour has, very sadly, been diagnosed with MND. Helping to care for her, I have seen first-hand the progression of her disease and her emotional struggle with loss of independence. This experience has shown me the limitations of modern medicine, and taught me the importance of accepting human mortality.

As a youth support leader with St John Ambulance, I helped to organise and deliver Cadet sessions which improved my leadership and teamwork skills. This built on skills that I had gained during my work as a Residential Counsellor with LINES Language Summer School, where I learnt how to relate to individuals from different cultures. Helping young people who were often feeling homesick taught me how acting with empathy and understanding helps make the best of any situation. It interested me to read a *BMJ* article saying that empathy is vital to being a good doctor, but overexposure to pain and suffering can cause empathy to decrease. I feel that it is not always easy to learn from difficult and painful situations, however it is essential to share and reflect on our experiences of suffering so we can improve our empathy.

I have played the piano for 15 years, and have successfully taken my grade 5 and practical musicianship. I now play for relaxation and enjoy the challenge of learning new pieces.

WARNING!

Do not write any of the above passages in your personal statement, as admissions tutors are all too aware of the existence of this book. They also use plagiarism software to determine similarities between scripts. Ensure that your personal statement is not only personal to you, but also honest.

'All I really want to see is a student has a determination to succeed and one who has researched everything about the career path they are looking to undertake. Evidence is king, to misquote another saying. Remember that the person reading the personal statement has read hundreds, in some cases thousands of them before and therefore will be able to distinguish between what is real and what is embellished. Keep it interesting but above all else, keep it personal. Be truthful to why you want to study the course and what you have done about researching that. Remember the value of work experience is to educate and inform and confirm to you that this path is the one you want to take. Oh and don't swallow a thesaurus! Understand each word you write. Communication is the hallmark of a good doctor.'

Advice from an admissions tutor

6 | The interview process

Once you've submitted your UCAS application, you must wait to hear from each of the universities you have applied to. If you meet or surpass their entry criteria, they may call you for interview. The universities use interviews to find out first hand whether the picture painted by your application is accurate and to investigate whether you have the skills necessary to become a successful medical practitioner.

Interviews for medical school usually take place between December and March each application cycle. While the thought of attending an interview can be somewhat scary, with careful preparation and practice it can ultimately turn out to be a rewarding experience.

Due to the impact of Covid-19, most universities went through a period of conducting interviews online. However, at the time of writing, most universities have returned to conducting face-to-face interviews. This situation is likely to continue to develop each year, so it is important to pay attention to the most up-to-date guidance from each university. Regardless of whether an interview occurs online or in person, the general principles remain the same, and so there is no difference in the preparation that needs to be carried out.

In this chapter, we will consider both multiple mini interviews (MMIs) and panel interviews, and the specific steps you will need to go through in order to prepare yourself, as well as more general interview pointers. Most of this guidance will be relevant to both types of interview and give appropriate general interview advice, but differences will be highlighted where necessary.

Making your interview a success

If you are invited to an interview, you need to prepare thoroughly for it, as you will not be given a second chance if you do not perform well. As with most other activities, the more you prepare and practise, the better your chance of success. Interviews can be stressful and you will be nervous, and so practice interviews are an important part of your preparation.

In this chapter, we look at common types of interview question and provide you with suggestions about how to approach them. You can then practise using the list of sample interview questions.

The questions that we look at in this chapter have all been asked at medical school interviews over recent years, and have been provided by students who have been interviewed and by members of medical school interview panels. You cannot always prepare for the odd, unpredictable questions that are bound to crop up, but the interviewers are not trying to catch you out, and they can be relied on to ask questions based on most of the general themes that are discussed here.

For most questions, there is not a single 'correct' answer, and, even if there were, you shouldn't try to memorise them and repeat them as you would lines in a theatre script. The purpose of presenting these questions, and some strategies for answering them, is to help you think about your answers before the interview and to enable you to put forward your own views clearly and with confidence.

When you have read through this section, and thought about the questions, arrange for someone to sit down with you and take you through the mock interview questions. (You might find it helpful to record the interview for later analysis.)

In general, interviewers are looking for intelligent students who have a good background knowledge of the world of medicine and healthcare. They are looking for individuals who have a desire to be a lifelong learner with an innate empathy and capacity to care for individuals. Interviews are the best way for universities to ascertain whether a student has the right blend of knowledge and skills and, as such, remain a vital component in the admissions process.

Multiple mini interviews (MMIs) versus panel interviews

In the past, the vast majority of medical interviews were panel-based, where two or more interviewers ask applicants a series of questions in a similar fashion to a traditional job interview. However, in recent years, most universities have moved towards multiple mini interviews (MMIs).

The MMI is designed to judge the suitability of a candidate to study medicine, and is felt to give a more accurate indication of potential academic performance during the course. This style of interview will have some similarities with the panel interview; however, the major difference is that applicants participate in a number of small interviews and tasks rather than just a single interview. The MMI at the University of Birmingham, for example, currently consists of six or seven eight-minute mini interview stations; these stations consist of a mix of interviews, role play and calculation tasks. It is important that you pay close attention to the instructions given to you in advance about the format of the interview, as well as the details given to you at each station so that you know exactly what is expected of you.

There are two main reasons for medical schools using this type of interview. Firstly, research has suggested that traditional panel interviews give a poor indication of the likely performance of the interviewee as an undergraduate; the MMI improves on this. Secondly, one of the major criticisms of the panel interview is that students can be heavily coached on the vast majority of question types and, as a result, do not give an accurate indication of their personality and character attributes. MMIs are therefore specifically designed to test those attributes of the interviewee that are unlikely to be improved by participating in preparation courses. They thereby allow the medical school to build a truer picture of what each candidate is like. Typical panel interviews have evolved somewhat in recent years and now tend to include a range of different tasks, albeit administered by the same panel of people, so they now more closely mimic what an MMI is designed to do.

Some universities are relatively tight-lipped about the exact detail of their interviews and give little information to the interviewees, while others are more open to sharing the details of exactly what will be faced. Queen's University Belfast gives detailed exemplar material and short tutorial video clips illustrating what will be faced at each station (visit www.qub.ac.uk/schools/mdbs/Study/Medicine/HowtoApply/MMIs).

The stations are carefully designed to assess attributes such as:

- compassion and empathy
- initiative and resilience
- interpersonal and communication skills
- organisational and problem-solving skills, decision making and critical thinking
- team working
- insight and integrity.

In order to prepare for either type of interview it is a good idea to ask multiple members of staff at your school, family and friends to ask you different questions and get you to think on your feet.

Typical interview themes and how to handle them (for both panel and MMI)

Although some of these questions will come up directly in some interviews, there will not be time to be asked all of them explicitly. Nevertheless, it is still essential to consider and prepare responses to all of them as they will provide a solid foundation of ideas that you can use for questions that pick up on similar themes.

1. Why do you want to become a doctor?

This is the question that is most likely to come up in one form or another and, as such, tends to be the most over-rehearsed one by applicants. There are no correct and incorrect answers to this question, but some areas to avoid include the following.

- One of my parents is a doctor and I want to be like them.
- The money's good and unemployment among doctors is low.
- The careers teacher told me to apply.
- It's glamorous.
- I want to join a respected profession, so it is either this or law.

Try answering the question now. Most sixth-formers find it quite hard to respond and are often not sure why they want to be a doctor. The interviewers will be sympathetic, but they do require a convincing answer. If you are struggling with this question, consider some of the approaches suggested below.

The story (option A)

You tell the interesting (and true) story of how your interest in medicine started, how you have made an effort to find out what is involved by undertaking work experience, and how this long-term and deep-seated interest has now become something of a passion. With this option, be prepared to back up your general statements with specific experiences from your placements.

The story (option B)

You tell the interesting (and true) story of how you, or a close relative, suffered from an illness that brought you into contact with the medical profession. This experience made you think of becoming a doctor and, since then, you have made an effort to find out what is involved … (as before).

The logical elimination of alternatives (option C)

In this approach you have analysed your career options and decided that you want to spend your life in a scientific environment (you have enjoyed science at school) but would find pure research too impersonal. Therefore, the idea of a career that combines the excitement of scientific investigation with a great deal of human contact is attractive. Since discovering that medicine offers this combination, you have investigated it (and other alternatives) thoroughly (visits to hospitals, GPs, etc.) and have become passionately committed to your decision.

The problems with this approach are that:

- they will have heard it all before
- you will find it harder to convince them of your passion for medicine as it can seem quite a cold way to choose a career.

Fascination with people (option D)

Some applicants can honestly claim to have a real interest in people and feel that a career in medicine would give them an opportunity to develop this. When coupled with an interest in biology, this can be a compelling argument due to the well-developed people skills that a successful doctor must have.

Answer with conviction

Your answer must be well considered and convincing, sound natural and not be over-rehearsed. Although an interview is a formal process, the more relaxed and natural your tone is, the better your chances are of success. Bear in mind that most of your interviewers will be doctors, and they (hopefully) will have chosen medicine because they, like you, had a burning desire to do so. Statements (as long as they are supported by evidence of practical research) such as 'and the more work I did at St James's, the more I realised that medicine is what I desperately want to do' are quite acceptable and far more convincing than saying 'medicine is the only career that combines science and the chance to work with people', because it isn't!

> 'The candidates who do best are those who are able to find something to be a good stress relief for them as the course can be quite overwhelming, from the interview process through to the job. We are looking for students who can balance their time so they do not burn out. In terms of an application, they need to be a reflective learner and to work out what kind of doctor they want to be, as this will affect the way they approach the degree. There is no substitute to life experience, and we are looking for candidates who can bring themselves to both the interview and the job. Be confident and assured when you are at the interview; we are friendly and just want to get the best out of you, not make you so nervous you cannot even answer the questions. Try and enjoy the experience.'
>
> *Advice from an admissions tutor*

2. What have you done to show your commitment to medicine and to the community?

This should tie in with your UCAS application. Your answer should demonstrate that you have a genuine interest in helping others. Ideally, you will have a track record of regular visits to your local hospital or hospice, where you will have had interactions with patients and staff and seen the less attractive side of patient care (such as cleaning bedpans). Acceptable alternatives are regular visits to an elderly person to do their chores, or volunteering for charities that care for disadvantaged groups. It is important that you can give details of experience that you have had while carrying out these placements in order to show that they are genuine and that you have taken time to reflect on what you have seen.

It isn't sufficient on its own to have just worked in a laboratory, out of sight of patients, or to have done so little work as to be trivial: 'I once walked around the ward of the local hospital.' While these experiences can be useful and valuable, they need to be backed up with experience of working with people, ideally in a clinical setting.

You also need to ask yourself why admissions tutors ask about work experience. It is not a tick-box exercise, rather they want to know whether you were there in body only, or if you were genuinely engaged with what was happening around you.

3. Why have you applied to this medical school?

Areas to avoid are:

- it has a good reputation (without giving specific, researched reasons)
- my father studied here
- it is close to the city's nightclubs.

Some of the reasons that you might have are given below.

- **Talking to people.** You have made a thorough investigation of a number of the medical schools that you have considered, by talking to your teachers, doctors and medical students you encountered during your work experience, and current students. They have given you a good picture of what it would be like to study here and have all said that university, course and style of teaching would suit you perfectly.
- **The course.** You have read the course details and feel that it is structured in a way that suits your style of study and medical interests. You like the fact that it is integrated/traditional/PBL/CBL/TBL and that students are brought into contact with patients at an early stage. Another related reason might be that you are attracted by the subject-based or systems-based teaching approach.
- **The open day.** You visited a number of medical schools' open days (either in person or virtually) and this one was by far the most interesting and informative. While attending, you talked to current medical students. You have spoken to the admissions tutor about your particular situation and asked their advice about suitable work experience, and he or she was particularly encouraging and helpful. You feel that the general atmosphere is one you would love to be part of.
- **The town/city/area.** Although you want to avoid discussing the nightlife or social scene, it is perfectly acceptable to talk about aspects of the local area that appeal to you.

> 'Treat the additional questionnaire and any written correspondence as though they have the same importance as the exams and the aptitude tests. Any time the university asks for information, it is because they are seriously considering your application and therefore any half-hearted efforts will not be viewed favourably by the department. Simply call it good practice in diligence for the profession.'
>
> *Advice from an admissions tutor*

4. Questions designed to assess your knowledge of the world of medicine

No one expects you to know all about your future career before you start at medical school, but they do expect you to have made an effort to find out something about it. If you are really interested in medicine, you will have a reasonable idea of common illnesses and diseases, and you will be aware of topical issues through your wider reading and research. The questions aimed at testing your knowledge of medicine can be broadly divided into five areas:

i. major medical issues
ii. the medical profession
iii. the National Health Service and funding health
iv. private medicine
v. ethical questions.

> 'The purpose of the interview is not to intimidate you, it is to get you to tell us why this is what you want above all else and what you have learnt. If we invite you to interview, you need to remember that it is because you have already jumped over a number of hurdles where many will have stumbled, and you are being seriously considered for a place at the medical school. This should give you a certain amount of confidence and hopefully allow you to enjoy the experience. Remember to maintain eye contact and body language throughout the interview, if you don't know the answer you can ask for clarification; however, try to give it a go; we will re-direct your answer if we need to and, most importantly, stick to what you know and not what you have *not* done please. We enjoy the interview process as meeting so many candidates from different backgrounds is the best part of this job. If you have any questions in advance, do not hesitate to contact the Admissions department – we can be friendly, despite the myth.'
>
> *Advice from an admissions tutor*

i. Major medical issues

The interviewers will expect you to be interested in medicine and to have a general awareness of current issues and new treatments. The best way to develop your understanding of these is to regularly read news articles and keep a file of the ones of interest to you and take the time to reflect on and record the illnesses and treatments that you came across during your work experience placements.

Keep a record of what you have read

Make sure that you read *New Scientist*, *Student BMJ* and, on a daily basis, a high-quality newspaper, news website or news app, that has a health or medical section. The *Independent* has excellent coverage of current health issues, and the *Guardian*'s health section is interesting and informative. Newspapers' websites often group articles thematically, which can save time. Taking as little as five minutes each day to read the most topical health news will ultimately have a major impact on developing your understanding. Make sure you keep a note of what you have read, and where and when you read it. You should also record any overall thoughts or impressions about what you have read. This will make it easier to find those interesting articles when you are preparing for an interview.

Topical illnesses

At any one time, the media tend to concentrate on one or two topical diseases which dominate coverage for a short period before fading into the background. Over the last 30 years, Ebola, CJD, SARS, bird flu, swine flu and Zika among others, resulted in relatively small numbers of deaths, even though they dominated the news at the time. Recently, illnesses such as Strep A, Mpox and Covid-19 have dominated the news headlines. As there has been so much media coverage of Covid-19, there will be no excuse for not having a solid understanding of the virus, its effects and its legacy across the globe.

While some of these diseases may not have a significant and lasting impact, they are often interesting in scientific terms, and the fact that they have been discussed in the media makes it likely that they will come up at interview. More details of the most relevant diseases are contained in Chapter 7.

The global picture

You may well be asked about what is happening on a global scale. You should know about the biggest killers (infectious diseases and circulatory diseases), trends in population changes, the role of the World Health Organization (WHO), and the differences in medical treatments between developed and developing countries. You can read more about this in Chapter 7.

TIP!

When discussing medical topics, try to use the correct terminology. If you are discussing a topic, do not be put off if you are not sure of the exact technical terms. It is better to show that you have a general grasp of an issue, even if it is not to the highest level of understanding.

ii. The medical profession

Although having a well-developed knowledge of health and disease is important, it is also vital to have an understanding of the medical profession and what being a doctor entails.

Questions in this area tend to relate to your understanding of the skills and attributes that a doctor needs. Good starting points for developing your understanding of the career are the BMA website, which has extensive guidance (www.bma.org.uk/advice-and-support/studying-medicine), and the GMC website, which has the 'Outcomes for Graduates' document (www.gmc-uk.org/education/standards-guidance-and-curricula/standards-and-outcomes/outcomes-for-graduates).

Begin by considering the importance of the technical skills that a doctor needs: the ability to carry out a thorough examination, to diagnose accurately and quickly what is wrong, and the skill to choose and organise the correct treatment and the precision to carry out treatment.

After this comes the ability to communicate effectively and sympathetically with the patient so that he or she can understand and participate in the treatment. The most important part of communication is listening.

Communication skills also have an important role to play in treatment – studies have shown that some patients get better more quickly when they feel involved and part of the medical team.

Other important skills include organisation, teamwork, empathy and working under pressure.

For each of these skills and the others that you identify, it is vital that you are prepared to discuss experiences from your life that illustrate that you have the skill or have taken steps to develop that skill. For example, you might say 'I was able to demonstrate my ability to work as part of a team during my Duke of Edinburgh expedition when I …'

Also make sure that you can define each skill. A good example of this is from an interview at Brighton and Sussex Medical School, where a student was asked to explain what empathy was and to distinguish it from sympathy.

iii. The National Health Service and funding health

With issues relating to the NHS dominating so much of the news, it is vital that you have a clear picture of the issues it faces. This will allow you to deal with any questions or scenarios that arise in relation to this in an interview.

An application to a medical school is also an application for a job, and you should have taken the trouble to find out something about your likely future employer. You should be aware of the structure of the NHS and the role that clinical commissioning groups and foundation trusts play. You need to know about the way in which doctors are trained, and the career paths that are open to medical graduates. When you are doing your work experience, you should take every opportunity to discuss the problems in the NHS with the doctors whom you meet. They will be able to give you first-hand accounts of what is happening, and this is an effective way of identifying the big issues that you can then go on to research further.

The key issues currently surrounding the NHS that should be investigated further are:

- the impact of NHS staff strikes and pay disputes
- the ongoing impact of the Covid-19 pandemic on the NHS
- funding
- staff shortages
- the social care crisis
- the cost of treating problems related to lifestyle diseases such as obesity
- caring for an ageing population
- steps being taken towards privatisation.

iv. Private medicine

Another area that needs careful thought concerns private medicine. Don't forget that many consultants have flourishing private practices and rely on private work for a major part of their income.

Most people agree that if you are run over by a bus you should be taken to hospital and treated at the taxpayers' expense. In general, urgent treatment for serious and life-threatening conditions should be provided by the NHS and we should all contribute towards its cost. On the other hand, most of us would agree that someone who wants cosmetic surgery for purely aesthetic reasons should pay for the operation themselves.

Having established these two extremes, one is left to argue about the point where the two systems meet. Should there be a firm dividing line between where both the NHS and private medicine operate? A good example of this is related to the provision of surgery for joint replacement. Most hip replacement operations are not a matter of life-or-death so should they be provided on the NHS, even if there is massive demand for them due to the ageing population of the UK? Or should they only be provided privately due to the limited resources of the NHS? Currently, there are strict criteria for referrals for this surgery and very long waiting lists, which effectively mean that this treatment is rationed.

You could also point out that private medicine does not necessarily harm the NHS. For example, the NHS has a problem of waiting lists. If 10 people are standing in a queue for a bus, everyone benefits if four of those waiting jump into a taxi – providing, of course, that they don't persuade the bus driver to drive it!

v. Ethical questions

Medical ethics is a fascinating area of moral philosophy. You won't be expected to answer questions on the finer points of philosophy, but many questions, scenarios and role plays in interviews will have their basis in medical ethics.

With ethical-based questions, you are most likely to be presented with a scenario, asked what issues it raises and what you would do in the situation. These are likely to include some elements directly related to medicine, but can sometimes be based on a purely non-medical situation. A non-medical example is a good place to start when considering how to deal with these questions. For example:

You see your friend stealing from a supermarket – what do you do?

The first thing to remember is that these questions are designed to assess a number of things:

- your understanding of moral issues
- whether you can look at problems from different angles
- your ability to weigh up arguments and come to a conclusion
- your knowledge of medical ethics.

When responding to this type of question, you should consider each of the following:

The context

Often, these scenarios are very limited on the detail they offer. Asking questions that would enable you to gather further information is a good idea, as it shows your ability to use questions to further your understanding. It is often the case that the interviewer won't provide much more detail, but posing these questions out loud shows your engagement with the scenario. Make sure you look at any clues in the scenario itself to try and learn more about the context of the situation, as this will shape how you deal with it. For example:

- who is involved?
- where is this scenario taking place?
- what is your role in the scenario?

The basics

Although ethical scenarios can raise a range of complex issues to consider, don't forget to mention the absolute basics of dealing with any situation, such as how you would communicate with the individuals involved and demonstrating empathy and compassion. This is a good opportunity to show that you know how to treat people with respect in difficult circumstances.

The difficulties with dealing with the scenario

These scenarios are not just about providing a solution to a problem, they are designed to see if you can identify the key challenges that you might face. Expressing the potential challenges that are posed is a good way of demonstrating your awareness, before you launch into trying to provide solutions. For example, in the example scenario about the friend stealing from the supermarket, it would be worth expressing that as the scenario involves a friend it would be more difficult to deal with than if it involved a stranger.

The key moral principles raised

You are not expected to be a legal expert, but you should be able to identify issues in the scenario that show you have an inbuilt understanding of right and wrong. In the example scenario, you would need to demonstrate that you understand that stealing is a crime, regardless of other influences.

The key principles of medical ethics

The bulk of your response to a medically based ethical scenario will be based around the key principles of medical ethics, but these can also be useful for non-medical related scenarios. There are many useful resources to help you understand these points, for example, the BMA Ethics toolkit, which can be found at www.bma.org.uk/advice-and-support/ethics/medical-students/ethics-toolkit-for-medical-students. You should take the time to read and understand each of the sections, as they will form the foundation of your response to any scenario, even if it's not medically based. It is impossible that one scenario will relate to all areas of medical ethics, so it is important that you identify the areas that are best suited to each scenario and discuss these in context.

Discussing the relevant ethical issues one-by-one will also help structure your overall response.

The four key pillars of medical ethics to consider are as follows:

- Non-maleficence – do no harm to the patient
- Beneficence – doing the most good for the patient
- Autonomy – the ability of the patient to choose
- Justice – upholding the law and fairness to all involved.

In addition to these four key pillars, issues such as consent, capacity and confidentiality are frequently relevant; the BMA Ethics toolkit discusses these further.

Providing a balanced argument

It is important that you show understanding of the situation from a range of perspectives, and don't jump to your own personal conclusions early on in your response.

Think about the views of the different people involved in the scenario, what they might be thinking and what they might do. It is important to note that you don't have to agree with a viewpoint in order to express it; you are just trying to signpost that you are aware of what the different perspectives are. A good example of this would be a scenario about somebody refusing to be vaccinated. You may be strongly pro-vaccination, yet would need to express an understanding of why someone might have differing opinions to both you and a healthcare professional.

In the example scenario, you would need to demonstrate that you are aware that it is wrong for your friend to steal, so something would need to be done; but at the same time show that you are aware of the difficulties that you might face as a result of confronting your friend. You could also demonstrate that you understand the perspective of the supermarket.

At the end of the scenario, you may want to add your own personal opinion or a firm conclusion. If so, make sure that this is done in a balanced and reasonable way, and only after you have outlined the different perspectives.

Your own relevant experience

If you have had first-hand experience of dealing with any of the issues that come up in a scenario, it can be useful to discuss this to illustrate how you would go about managing it. Don't worry if you don't have relevant experience, as it is highly unlikely that you will; just don't be afraid to use anything that is relevant.

5. Role plays and questions aimed at finding out whether you have the necessary skills to be a doctor

One of the reasons for interviewing you is to see whether you will fit successfully into both the medical school and the medical profession. The interviewers will try to find out if your views and approach to life are likely to make you an acceptable colleague in a profession that, to a great extent, depends on teamwork.

The vast majority of questions, regardless of what they are about, will have another important purpose: to assess your ability to communicate in a friendly and effective way with strangers even when under pressure. This skill will be very important when you come to deal with patients.

Increasingly common in interviews is the use of role play. The scenario you may be asked to act out may, but this is not guaranteed, have a medical basis, but will definitely not rely on your knowledge of science or first aid. This is to assess attributes such as communication, compassion and calmness under pressure. For example:

You are approached by your elderly neighbour, whose husband has just died. Your neighbour hasn't left her home in three months, but has an upcoming appointment at a hospital that is 20 miles away. She is anxious about attending the hospital appointment and is considering not going. How would you deal with this situation?

In this situation, you would be expected to start communicating with the widow to try and find out what their worries are, while at the same time reassuring them and trying to keep them calm. You could also suggest some solutions to the problem. Commonly, the person playing opposite you will act upset, angry or confused to see how you respond. It is worth trying to practise scenarios like these with friends or family members to get a feel for how you would react.

Another example:

You are reversing out of your driveway when you accidentally run over your neighbour's cat, although nobody else has seen you do it. You have to break the news to your neighbour. What do you do?

The interviewer is looking for evidence of the following:

- clear communication
- honesty
- a caring and empathetic attitude
- ability to successfully deal with a person who is upset or angry.

6. Questions about your UCAS application

The personal statement section, in which you write about yourself, is a fertile area for interviewers to base questions on. It is therefore vital to keep a copy of your personal statement so you can brush up on what you have written in advance of the interview.

If you have mentioned anything specific in your statement that is of interest to you, make sure that you can discuss it if asked. For example, if you have mentioned that you completed an EPQ based on the incidence and spread of avian flu, you should ensure that you can give an overview of your findings.

This is why it is particularly important to ensure that everything in your statement is truthful; anything that you have exaggerated or been untruthful about could potentially come back to haunt you at this point.

7. Questions about how you might contribute to the life of the medical school

These questions can come in many forms and could either focus on how you have contributed to your school or college in the past or how you intend to contribute to university life in the future.

The best approach is to give an answer that demonstrates that you understand the balance needed between study and extracurricular pursuits. However, this type of question is not usually designed to catch you out; it is often a genuine enquiry about whether you have a life beyond your studies and can relax as well as work hard.

You may find it helpful to know that, in one London medical school, the interviewers are told to ask themselves if the candidate has made good use of the opportunities available to them, and whether they have the personal qualities and interests appropriate to student life and a subsequent career in medicine. A lack of evidence of participation in life beyond the curriculum is unlikely to be a positive factor.

8. Unpredictable questions

Even with all of the preparation in the world, there is no way that every question or topic can be pre-empted. If you get asked a question that you have never considered before, try to think about the skills that they are trying to test. This can often help you to demystify the random question you have been given. Often in these scenarios, just being a generally nice, caring and thoughtful human being will help you to give a solid answer, even if you are unsure of the correct approach. Some examples of questions and scenarios are as follows.

- *If you won £20 million on the lottery, what would you do with it?*
- *Tell me about your family.*
- *You start discussing a medical issue with a patient, but they are more concerned about telling you about their washing machine that is broken. How do you deal with the situation?*

In each of these situations, make sure you stay calm and don't panic. If you panic, you are more likely to rush your answer and say something you don't mean. If the question has really surprised you, take a few seconds to plan the key ideas that you wish to discuss rather than just rushing straight into something. However, you still need to treat these questions as seriously as ones that are directly connected to medicine. Also make sure that you don't take offence at the fact that the interviewer is deviating from what you think should be happening in a medical interview; one student got quite aggressive in an interview because she thought she wasn't being asked the questions that she was expecting. Avoid this at all costs!

Although some degree of openness and honesty are useful for these sort of questions, make sure you avoid saying anything that is going to leave a negative impression. For example, telling the interviewer that you hate your family and spend all of your time arguing with them is not going to do anything to impress them, even if it is true!

Another question that interviewees always fear is being asked about something scientific or technical that they have never heard of. For example: 'What is the drug x used for?'

You are not expected to have the knowledge that a qualified doctor has and so you would only be asked this type of question if the drug in question had been in the news recently, or if you had mentioned something related to it in your personal statement. So your pre-interview preparation (making sure you are up to date with recent events and being familiar with your personal statement) will help you here.

This type of question can also be a way to see how you handle yourself in difficult situations and when put under stress. There may be no expectation that you will know about this topic and it might just be to see how your thought processes work or if you can synthesise ideas and information based on your general knowledge and understanding.

Your questions for the interviewers

In panel interviews you may get the opportunity to ask questions of the people who have interviewed you. Bear in mind that the interviews are carefully timed, and that your attempts to impress the panel with 'clever' questions may do quite the opposite. The golden rule is: only ask a question if you are genuinely interested in the answer (which, of course, you were unable to find during your careful reading of the prospectus and website). Some medical schools will not allow you to ask questions of the interviewing panel and it is extremely unlikely that you will be able to ask questions during an MMI. Questions can be asked of other staff or current students during the time you are there, but not in the interview itself.

Questions to avoid

- What is the structure of the first year of the course?
- Will I be able to live in halls of residence?
- When will I first have contact with patients?
- Can you tell me about the intercalated BSc option?

As well as being dull questions, the answers to these will be available in the prospectus and on the website, and you will show that you have obviously not done any serious research.

One final piece of advice on interviews: keep your answers relatively short and to the point. Nothing is more challenging for an interviewer than dealing with an answer that rambles on. Make sure your answer is detailed, but at the same time, don't be tempted to wander off into areas that don't relate to the question. If your answer does go on too long, expect to be abruptly interrupted; the interviewers aren't trying to be purposefully rude when they do this, but they do have limited time to get through all of the questions.

Mock interview questions

As explained at the beginning of the chapter, interview technique for both types of interview can be improved with practice. You can use this section of the book as a source of mock interview questions.

Remember that these questions are designed to develop your skills and give you practice in interview technique, rather than being questions to memorise the answers to.

Your motivation to study medicine

- Tell us about yourself.
- Why do you want to be a doctor? What do you want to achieve in medicine?
- What steps have you taken to try to find out whether you really do want to become a doctor? What do you think are the main challenges of becoming a doctor/studying medicine?
- What factors might be behind a student dropping out of medical school?
- How do you deal with stress?

Knowledge of the medical school and teaching methods

- What interests you about the curriculum at [medical school]?
- Tell us what attracts you most and least about [medical school].
- What do you know about problem-based learning?
- Why do you know about the approach to teaching at this medical school?
- Why do you think our style of teaching will suit you personally?

Depth and breadth of interest

- Do you read any medical publications?
- What do you think was the greatest public health advance of the twentieth century?
- Can you describe an interesting place you have been to (not necessarily medical) and explain why it was so?
- Share something that you have recently read related to the world of medicine that interested you.

Empathy

- Give an example of a situation where you have supported a friend in a difficult social circumstance. What issues did they face and how did you help them?
- How would you go about informing a patient that they have terminal cancer?
- What does the word empathy mean to you? How do you differentiate empathy from sympathy?
- Scenario: *You are a medical student, and a friend of yours tells you they are feeling anxious and stressed about upcoming exams.* How do you respond to this?
- What do you guess an overweight person might feel and think after being told their arthritis is due to their weight?
- A friend has asked your advice on how to tell her parents that she intends to drop out of university and go off travelling. How would you respond?

Teamwork

- Tell us about a team situation you have experienced. What did you learn about yourself and about successful team-working?
- Thinking about your membership of a team (in a work, sport, school or other setting), can you tell us about the most important contributions you made to the team?
- When you think about yourself working as a doctor, who do you think will be the most important people in the team you will be working with?
- Who are the important members of a multidisciplinary healthcare team? Why?
- Are you a leader or a follower?
- What are the advantages and disadvantages of being in a team? Do teams need leaders?

Personal insight

- Have you ever been in a situation where you realise afterwards that what you said or did was wrong? What did you do about it? What should you have done?
- How do you think doctors keep up to date with changes and advances during a long career?
- What are your outside interests and hobbies? Which do you think you will continue at university?
- Tell us two personal qualities you have that would make you a good doctor. Give an example of a situation in which you have demonstrated this quality.
- What would you say are your strengths? Give an example of when you demonstrated one of these strengths.
- Medical training is long and being a doctor can be stressful. Some doctors who qualify never practise. What makes you think you will stick to it?
- What do you think will be the most difficult things you might encounter during your training? How will you deal with them?
- How do you know when you are stressed?

Understanding of the role of medicine in society

- What problems are there in the NHS other than the lack of funding?
- Would you argue that medicine is a science or an art, and why?
- Why do you think we hear so much about doctors and the NHS in the media today?
- In what ways do you think doctors can promote good health, other than direct treatment of illness?
- Do you think patients' treatments should be limited by the NHS budget or do they have the right to new therapies no matter what the cost?
- What do you understand by the term 'alternative' medicine? Do you think it falls within the remit of the NHS?

Work experience

- What experiences have given you insight into the world of medicine? What have you learnt from these?
- What aspect of your work experience did you find the most challenging, and why?
- Share something from your work experience or voluntary work that particularly interested you.
- Share something from your work experience that particularly shocked you.
- What aspect of your work experience would you recommend to a friend thinking about medicine, and why?
- Thinking of your work experience, can you tell me about a difficult situation you have dealt with and what you learned from it?

Tolerance of ambiguity

- Should doctors have a role in contact sports such as boxing?
- Do you think doctors should ever go on strike?
- How do you think doctors should treat injury or illness due to self-harm, smoking or excess alcohol consumption?
- Female infertility treatment is expensive, has a very low success rate and is even less successful in smokers. To whom do you think it should be available?
- Would you prescribe the oral contraceptive pill to a 14-year-old girl who is having a sexual relationship with her boyfriend?

Ethical scenarios and role plays

For each of these situations, you may be asked to explain what you would do or be expected to act it out as part of a role play.

- *You are working in a café as a member of the waiting staff when a customer who is allergic to nuts brings their order back to you as they can see nuts in it.* How do you respond to the customer?
- *A friend tells you he feels bad because his family has always cheated to obtain extra benefits.* How would you respond?
- *A close friend has just split up with their partner. They are distraught and have expressed they are considering suicide.* How do you deal with the situation?
- *You are a medical student undertaking a placement at a GP clinic; during an appointment, the doctor is required to take an emergency phone call outside the room, and so asks you to take the patient's blood pressure while he is absent. Once the doctor has left, the patient begins to show discomfort and unease, and refuses to let you take their blood pressure.* How would you respond to the patient? How would you calm the patient? Why do you think the patient doesn't want you to take their blood pressure?
- *You are a first-year medical student who is part of a WhatsApp group with other medical students, one of whom is a third-year student called Oscar. Oscar has been frequently sending pictures of*

patients without any personal details, and has even been laughing and making fun of their maladies. After a while, you start to think that perhaps this isn't right, so you voice your concerns to the group. Most participants agree not to continue with the activity; however, Oscar says that you shouldn't be so worried and that everyone does it. Thus, he continues to send pictures of patients. Why are Oscar's actions wrong? How would you respond to Oscar?

Creativity, innovation and imagination

- *You are going to university and you can take a suitcase with just six items in it.* What would you take and why?
- You are provided with a needle and thread and asked to pick it up with surgical scissors; you then need to use the scissor-held needle to thread a pattern that is provided.
- Imagine a world in 200 years' time where doctors no longer exist. In what ways do you think they could be replaced?
- Is it better to give healthcare or aid to developing countries?
- Describe as many uses as you can for a mobile phone charger.
- How might you improve the process of selecting students for this medical school?
- *Your house catches fire in the night. You are told you can pick only one object to take with you when escaping.* What would it be and why?

Points for the interviewee to consider

In addition to your engagement with each question you are asked, it is vital that you give a generally good impression to your interviewers. You should consider these dos and don'ts.

Do

- Speak clearly and at an appropriate volume.
- Answer in a friendly and positive way.
- Maintain a good degree of eye contact.
- Dress smartly. Remember it is easy to remove clothing if you feel overdressed.

For online interviews, well in advance, check the following:

- the device you will be using has a good-quality camera and micro-phone
- there is a good internet connection where you will be conducting the interview
- the background is appropriate for an interview situation.

Don't

- Exhibit body language tics, such as tapping your fingers on the table.
- Wear overpowering aftershave or perfume.

- Slouch in the chair.
- Swear.

You should dress smartly and sensibly for your interview, in the same way that you would for a job interview, but you should also feel comfortable.

Your aim must be to give an impression of good personal organisation and cleanliness. Make a particular point of your hair and fingernails – you never see a doctor with dirty fingernails. Always polish your shoes before an interview, as this type of detail will be noticed. Don't go in smelling strongly of aftershave, perfume or food. Make sure that you arrive early and are well prepared for the interview.

Try to achieve eye contact with each member of the panel and, as much as possible, address your answer directly to the panel member who asked the question (glancing regularly at the others), not up in the air or to a piece of furniture. Most importantly, try to relax and enjoy the interview. This will help you to project an open, cheerful personality.

Finally, watch out for irritating mannerisms. These are easily checked if you record footage of a mock interview on your phone. The interviewers will not listen to what you are saying if they are all watching to see when you are next going to scratch your left ear with your right thumb!

The interviewers

The interviewers can come from a wide variety of backgrounds, but it is likely that some of them will be academic staff from the medical school. They are often joined by medical students, practising doctors and sometimes members of the public. All interviewers are trained to apply the interview criteria accurately and fairly.

While you can expect the interviewers to be friendly, it is possible that at least one of them may come across as aggressive, angry or disinterested. Don't be put off by this; it is either an interview technique that the interviewer has been asked to adopt, or just the natural personality of the interviewer. Either way, stay positive and calm and don't deviate from how you would normally behave.

Questionnaires

An increasing number of medical schools have started to use additional forms for students to fill in with details of their work experience and personal skills. It is important to treat this even more seriously than your personal statement as it is likely to have even closer scrutiny.

A good example of this type of form is from the University of Manchester, which uses an online portal to collect information about your non-academic pursuits. This is structured in the following sections.

- Experience in a caring role.
- Hobbies and interests.
- Team working.
- Motivation for medicine.
- Why Manchester?

Source: www.bmh.manchester.ac.uk/study/medicine/apply/non-academic

Although it is likely that you will use experiences from your personal statement in these sections, it is important that they are written from scratch and not just copied straight over.

What happens next?

If your interview score is below the threshold score but close to it, you may be put on an official or unofficial waiting list. If you are offered a place, you will receive correspondence from the medical school telling you what you need to achieve in your A levels: this is called a conditional offer. In addition, the conditions of your offer will be added to UCAS Track, although this can take a little bit of time, so don't worry if you are made to wait a short while. Post-A level students who have achieved the necessary grades will usually be given unconditional offers in terms of the academic requirements, but may still be made conditional offers in relation to criminal record and health checks. If your application is not successful, all you will get is a notification from UCAS saying that you have been rejected. If this happens, it is not necessarily the end of the road in medicine, as you may be able to reapply as a post-A level applicant. What you must do in this situation is contact the universities that you applied to and ask for feedback about why you were unsuccessful. However, be warned, some universities don't give feedback, while others provide seemingly random comments that seem to bear no resemblance to your memory of the interview. Some universities will be more helpful than others and give relatively detailed feedback, which will give you points to consider.

Case study

Camrun is a second-year medical student at the University of Exeter. He arrived at his decision to study medicine following his voluntary work in Cambodia.

'I decided to study medicine after working at Khmer Sight, an ophthalmic charity based in Cambodia, for about four months. This, alongside my work experience placement at Birmingham Children's Hospital, reinforced my desire to pursue a career in medicine.

'Both of these experiences taught me how hectic and stressful medicine can be, but also how incredibly rewarding it is. Working in both Asia and the UK gave me a great insight into how the different healthcare systems work, and how grateful people can be when healthcare isn't guaranteed. I also gained some useful clinical knowledge, especially in the context of eyes.

'During my first year, I was quite surprised that medical schools take a much less active role in your learning than I was familiar with. This was especially true in clinical skills, where you are taught something and then left to your own devices to practise it and maintain a high level of proficiency, which can be quite daunting but allows you to learn quickly!

'I find the clinical aspects of the course the most interesting. In general, I have always preferred subjects that are more applied and practical than just learning the factual and theoretical side of things. There are some heavy expectations placed on you for some parts of the course, especially adapting to new styles of learning and assessment quickly, such as the Objective Structured Clinical Examinations (OSCEs), though you do so many of them over the course of the degree that you get used to them quickly. This style of learning parallels medicine and gets you used to thinking on your feet, as nothing in medicine is certain. I have really enjoyed my placements to date, and everyone is very eager to help you learn.

'At the moment, I'm not sure what I would like to specialise in. There are lots of options and I think through further placements, I will gain more insight into the possible routes for me.

'My advice for students aspiring to study medicine is not to rush into it, even if that means taking a gap year to make absolutely sure it is for you. I know for certain I wouldn't have enjoyed the course at 18 years old, but taking some time out allowed me to reflect on whether it was the right course for me, so I was more prepared when I did begin studying several years later. Lots of people feel demoralised when they are rejected during the application process, but you shouldn't let this deter you from trying. When I applied, I received a number of rejections, but managed to secure a place at Exeter. Don't worry about rejections and don't be too proud to take some time out to better yourself so you can improve your application next time around. I would also encourage applicants to practise as much as they can for UCAT, as a high score can really help with getting interviews.'

7 | Current issues

It is obviously impossible to know about all illnesses and issues in medicine. However, being aware of some of the issues in medicine today will be of enormous benefit, particularly if you are asked, as many candidates are, to extrapolate and elucidate on 'an issue' in an interview. Showing that you have an awareness of issues on more than a passing or superficial level demonstrates intelligence, interest and enthusiasm for medicine.

This will undoubtedly stand you in good stead next to a candidate who either is very hazy or is at worst completely unaware of a major issue in medicine. The following section illustrates, albeit briefly, some of the major issues that are currently causing debate, both in medical circles and in wider society. A little bit of awareness and knowledge can go a long way to securing and leaving a positive impression on an interview panel.

National Health Service (NHS)

Since its initiation in 1948, the NHS has undergone major reforms to improve the services it provides. However, it has become a victim of its own success. No one can deny there are problems; however, a lot of these are because the NHS has got better at helping people, raising expectations and, perhaps unfairly, the service is judged on that. The state of the NHS is a very topical issue, and is therefore a very common area of questioning by interview teams.

Structure of the NHS

In England, the NHS comprises a number of core organisations.

- The Department of Health and Social Care is the government department responsible for the distribution of funding for health and social care in England, as well as policy making.
- NHS England is an independent body that is not under government control. It is responsible for improving healthcare outcomes and determining the priorities of the NHS. It is also responsible for commissioning primary care services.
- Clinical Commissioning Groups (CCGs) are statutory NHS bodies run by clinical staff, such as GPs, nurses and consultants. They play a significant role in their local area, where they commission

necessary healthcare and acquire the appropriate funding. In this way, they are responsible for around 60% of the NHS budget.

NHS funding

Since the 1980s, it has been evident that as scientific advances occurred, the cost of the services provided by the NHS would continue to increase. The majority of news stories and the negativity that surrounds the NHS often come down to its chronic underfunding. In recent years, some dramatic changes have occurred in a bid to limit these pressures.

Privatisation of the NHS

From 2012, NHS hospitals were allowed to cap their private work to 49% (previous to this, the cap had been much lower), and NHS trusts could become self-governing by 2014. However, by September 2014, figures published showed that the NHS was nearly £1 billion in debt. External governing bodies stepped in to alleviate the accrued debt, but there was concern that focusing on profits could destabilise local hospitals. The Covid-19 pandemic has changed the landscape of healthcare in the UK, and with the increased demands on its already limited resources, further privatisation is a possibility.

Things to consider

Most people will automatically oppose privatisation of the NHS, as they see it as a detraction from one of the NHS's core principles: free healthcare at the point of use. There are some arguments surrounding privatisation, and it is worth you familiarising yourself with them. You might want to consider the following.

- Fairness – privatisation of the NHS may ultimately result in some provisions only being available to those able to afford them.
- Feasibility – when the NHS was introduced, the consequences of an ageing population were not considered, and it is now simply too expensive to run as it stands.
- Efficiency – when compared to insurance-based health programmes that are privately run, such as those in the US, publicly funded healthcare systems are far more efficient in that considerably less money is spent per person.
- Continuity – in some cases, continuity of care is required, or at least preferred, and this may not always be possible in privatised sectors.
- Costs – in private healthcare, drugs and other medical interventions have varying costs, and they typically increase year on year.
- Choices – it is possible that privatisation may lead to enhanced options regarding where a patient is treated and what that treatment might be. However, it is unlikely that such choice would be available at an equal level, and may be of greater benefit to those who are able to afford it.

Recent changes within the NHS

> *'Reforms so big they can be seen from space.'*
>
> *Former NHS Chief Executive Sir David Nicholson*

Recent history of the NHS

In 2018, the NHS celebrated its 70-year anniversary, during which time medicine had been revolutionised with regard to innovation and care. Clinical outcomes were better, cancer survival rates were higher and the number of clinical commissioning groups (20 in total) moving out of special measures and improving was positive.

Nevertheless, pressures on the NHS were greater than ever in 2017. The previous budget had not provided enough money for all of the NHS departments and the Secretary of State for Health Jeremy Hunt's divisive order to NHS bosses to continue with current waiting times was, within the service, considered unsustainable. The NHS itself in 2017 stated that it was confronting certain paradoxes.

- '*We're getting healthier, but we're using the NHS more*'. It was estimated that life expectancy had been rising by five hours a day, but alongside that the need for NHS care was more pronounced. This was largely due to the growing and ageing population, with more than half a million more people aged over 75 since 2010 and an estimated two million more by 2020.
- '*The quality of NHS care is demonstrably improving, but we're becoming far more transparent about care gaps and mistakes*'. Survival rates were better but this had raised public expectations.
- '*Staff numbers are up, but staff are under greater pressure*'. There were 8,000 more doctors and nurses working in the NHS than there were in 2014, but these staff were not spread across all departments, rather they were clustered within certain specialisms.
- '*The public are highly satisfied with the NHS, but concerned for its future*'. Independent data from the last three decades showed that the level of satisfaction and trust from the public with the NHS was at one of its highest peaks in 2017.

The NHS Five Year Forward View described three improvement opportunities: a health gap, a quality gap, and a financial sustainability gap.

Improvements made in 2017 included:

- action on prevention and public health
- plain packaging for cigarettes
- national diabetes prevention programme
- sugar tax agreed to reduce childhood obesity
- vaccination of over 1 million infants against meningitis and an additional 2 million children against flu
- public health campaigns such as 'Be Clear on Cancer' and 'Act Fast'.

The NHS Five Year Forward View has made a positive impact on society's healthcare standards. NHS England has now written a plan, following the 70th birthday of the NHS in 2018, to sustain it for at least another decade – this is the Long Term Plan. The Long Term Plan has a greater focus on prevention over cure, and greater access to out of hours GPs and urgent care services. In summary, the Long Term Plan aims to:

- improve provision of care based on the needs of the individual patient
- improve the quality of care at GP level to reduce hospital admissions
- improve accessibility of treatment, with faster access to services and treatments and improved proximity to patients' homes
- provide online GP consultations
- improve education of patients with diseases such as diabetes, so that they can more effectively self-manage
- invest in cancer interventions, with a greater emphasis on early diagnosis for better prognostic outcomes
- increase the number of nursing undergraduate places at university.

Perhaps one of the most exciting prospects of the Long Term Plan is an accessible and rapid screening mechanism for heart disease, which is the largest global cause of mortality. This will be achieved using risk stratification, whereby patients presenting with potential risk factors, such as diabetes, high blood pressure, atrial fibrillation or even family history of cardiovascular disease, are identified and interventions are put in place. These interventions will be largely based around changes to lifestyle, though some medical interventions, such as introduction to an anticoagulation medication, may also be utilised. The main idea behind the screening process is to reduce disease progression, as well as the associated complications of treating more advanced disease; more targeted use of resources in a specialised manner; assisting patients with informed decision-making regarding their lifestyle choices; and, overall, to reduce mortality rates through early intervention. The most up to date information about the NHS's Long Term Plan can be found at www.longtermplan.nhs.uk.

The NHS is ever-changing and it is impacted by a wide range of factors. It is crucial that you keep a close eye on things relating to the NHS in the news, including regulatory and structural changes, and new findings relating to specific aspects of health. Some of the most current issues at the time of writing are discussed below.

Strike action

Throughout 2023, junior doctors and consultants took industrial action and took part in a number of strikes. Throughout the strikes, emergency cover was still provided, but there was some disruption to pre-booked, non-urgent treatments, such as outpatient procedures.

The strikes that took place in October 2023 were the sixth by junior doctors and the third by consultants, and it was the first time in the history of the NHS that both groups of doctors went on strike simultaneously. The strikes have been organised as a consequence of insufficient pay, with both unions seeking above-inflation pay rises amid a cost of living crisis. The joint strike action of junior doctors and consultants was coordinated to maximise effectiveness.

In late 2023, the recently appointed Secretary of State for Health Victoria Atkins and senior doctors reached a deal that they hoped would bring an end to strike action by consultants. However, at the time of going to press (January 2024), junior doctors were continuing to hold strike action.

Given the enormous impact that these strikes have had on patient care, they have been divisive among the general public, with general opinion being torn between frustration at what are regarded as well-paid individuals, who are aware of the jobs that they are entering into, daring to strike, and an appreciation and understanding of the extreme pressures that junior doctors face in an already stretched NHS.

The Covid-19 pandemic

The Covid-19 coronavirus pandemic influenced every aspect of our lives, with the NHS undoubtedly the most heavily impacted. It affected people's livelihoods, job security, incomes and social lives, all of which are required for healthy living.

The World Health Organization declared the outbreak of Covid-19 as a pandemic on 11 March 2020. The first cluster of cases of pneumonia with an unknown cause was reported in Wuhan City in the Hubei Province in China on 31 December 2019; the cause was identified as a novel coronavirus, SARS-Cov-2, causing the associated disease Covid-19, on 12 January 2020.

At the time of writing (September 2023), mass testing and reporting of positive cases has been largely abandoned, though there are estimated to have been over 771 million cases confirmed around the globe and almost 7 million deaths, which starkly illustrates the devastating impact of a novel infection within the human population.

The source of the outbreak is thought to be zoonotic – caused by an infectious pathogen that has transferred from a non-human animal to humans – though investigations are ongoing. After the initial cases in Wuhan, all subsequent cases have been due to human-to-human transmission which is the reason behind all of the protocols that soon became part of our daily lives – wearing face masks, remaining socially distanced and, at the peaks of infection, the country going into lockdown, where the government encouraged everyone to stay at home as much as was physically possible.

As soon as the Covid-19 outbreak was declared a pandemic, there was a mass shift in research funding and focus to efforts to prevent its transmission and to find a suitable treatment. Incredibly, as early as December 2020, the UK had embarked on a mass vaccination programme thanks to the approval of a vaccine developed by Pfizer and BioNtech. By January another vaccine developed by AstraZeneca was also approved for use in the UK's vaccination programme (see page 121).

Nevertheless, cases continued to increase as the virus mutated and new variants of concern emerged. The Delta variant had become dominant in the UK in June 2021, after first being detected in India in December 2020. As it was more infectious, it spread rapidly around the UK. In early December 2021, the Omicron variant emerged and was even more infectious than the Delta variant. Given the significant strain already on the NHS in the winter and the phenomenal rate at which the Omicron variant spread through the UK population, the UK government put out an urgent appeal calling for people to get their vaccines, reducing the time between first and second doses and second and booster doses, as well as encouraging people to work from home where possible.

In September 2023, the vast majority of restrictions have been lifted globally, with only guidance surrounding staying home if you are unwell and undertaking a test remaining in place. As such, normal life has largely resumed, though those at high risk are still advised to take additional precautions. Booster programmes are in place for the vaccine for those that are deemed to be clinically vulnerable, including those with health conditions and the elderly. The booster vaccinations are newer

The clinical features of Covid-19?

Perhaps one of the biggest problems with Covid-19 is its presentation: it varies considerably in terms of the symptoms that people experience, and those impacted can be completely asymptomatic or hospitalised.

The common symptoms include:

- fever
- new, continuous cough
- shortness of breath
- fatigue
- loss of appetite
- loss of taste and smell.

However, this list of symptoms is not exclusive, and people have also experienced sore throats, headaches, nasal congestion, diarrhoea, nausea and vomiting.

versions that protect against the most recently emerged strains, suggesting that moving forward, it will be managed in a similar way to influenza. As another winter approaches, concerns are beginning to increase again as another new variant emerges and cases rise, but with measures such as the booster vaccine in place to support the most vulnerable, the general population and healthcare providers are considerably less worried than they have been in previous years.

Lockdown

The first lockdown was called on 23 March 2020. It was strict and meant that individuals in the UK could only leave their homes for food, medication or to provide care for vulnerable individuals, as well as to undertake one form of exercise per day. This involved closure of schools (leading to online teaching), and even the cancellation of exams. Initially, the lockdown was only due to last for three weeks, but it was extended far beyond this, until 10 May. Another, slightly less strict lockdown was introduced in England on 5 November 2020 for four weeks, and then another strict lockdown began on 6 January 2021 and was gradually relaxed from 8 March, with all restrictions removed on 21 June 2021 until December 2021 when regional restrictions were introduced over the Christmas period.

So, why were lockdowns imposed?

- To stop the spread of infection.
- To prevent the NHS from becoming overwhelmed; in the initial lockdown it was also to provide time to prepare hospitals for further admissions by acquiring specialist equipment such as ventilators.
- To provide time for the development of treatment plans for those becoming more severely unwell.
- To allow time for the development of a track and trace system.

During the first lockdown, the NHS did become more equipped and significant efforts went into the development of Nightingale hospitals, which were set up as temporary Covid-19 hospitals. Though setting up additional hospitals specialised for treatment of a particular disease during a pandemic was fairly logical, the issue that emerged was a lack of staff. In existing hospitals, many specialist staff were redeployed to Covid wards, meaning that existing practices in a wide range of specialities were stretched enormously, negatively impacting patient care in these areas.

Impact of Covid-19 on the NHS

Covid-19 severely disrupted NHS provisions in the UK. Public health restrictions and measures were put in place to control the spread of the virus and protect the most vulnerable individuals in the population, but

Lockdown

Lockdowns proved effective in reducing cases, hospitalisations and deaths. However, there were negative consequences to th lockdowns.

- The economic consequences of lockdown were dire, with many people becoming unemployed.
- There were increases in reports of domestic abuse.
- Many people reported a decline in their mental health.
- School closures impacted ongoing student attainment and long-term attendance.
- Illnesses went undiagnosed due to individuals' reluctance to visit GP surgeries and hospitals during lockdown.

the reality is that this was done in the midst of continuous budget reductions for the NHS. As such, in order to support the increased demand on healthcare services, healthcare provision for non-Covid-19 patients was heavily scaled back.

The NHS entered the pandemic on the back foot – without enough beds and staff per capita across the country. Staffing shortages were also apparent prior to the onset of the virus. NHS trusts therefore had to make large-scale changes to their services to enhance the capacity for treating patients with Covid-19. As well as the redeployment of specialist staff, thousands of patients were discharged early to free up beds and non-urgent treatment was largely postponed. A high proportion of appointments were also postponed or moved online, which is thought to have led to many health issues requiring urgent attention being missed, or treatment interventions being made too late, having an enormous negative impact on patient health.

Throughout the first lockdown period, Accident and Emergency use and admissions dropped significantly enough to raise concerns. For example, the British Heart Foundation reported that there had been a 38% drop in emergency heart surgeries in London in the second half of March 2020, suggesting that patients stayed away for fear of contracting the virus and putting additional pressure on the NHS. NHS England were clear that cancer treatment must continue, but inevitable delays and disruption to surgery and chemotherapy would result in an increase in deaths. Of course, the impact didn't stop here – mental health, maternity services, routine immunisations in children and the management of chronic conditions are also thought to have suffered considerably.

Shielding

In order to protect the NHS, the most clinically vulnerable people were asked to shield by staying indoors and isolating entirely. Early data from the most affected countries, including China and Italy, indicated that fatalities from Covid-19 infections were more likely in those with underlying health conditions, including heart disease, lung disease and chronic obstructive pulmonary disease (COPD), diabetes and high blood pressure. Those identified as being most at risk were contacted by the NHS. By isolating, it was hoped that they were less likely to contract the virus and, as a result, the number of patients requiring treatment in intensive care would remain manageable.

Alarmingly, the Covid-19 deaths highlighted the disparities between the health of populations in different parts of the country. Not all elderly people, for example, were affected in the same way, and those living in more socially and economically deprived areas saw higher death rates. Similarly, there was a disproportionate impact on black, Asian and minority ethnic communities in the UK.

Despite Covid-19 persisting and cases remaining relatively high in the UK, the government officially ended shielding on 1 April 2021. The reasons for this were that, as a virus, Covid-19 was now better understood, a largely successful vaccine programme had been established, and that the restrictive nature of shielding on people's lives and wellbeing must be considered. Those considered to be extremely clinically vulnerable, such as the immunocompromised, were encouraged to take extra precautions as advised by their own healthcare specialists.

Future challenges

Even nearly four years after the onset of the pandemic in the UK, it is far from over. One of the initial major concerns was about the reinstatement of routine care. The NHS aims for a waiting time of no more than 18 weeks, yet before the virus had reached the UK, around 730,000 individuals had been on a waiting list for a longer duration than this for routine hospital appointments, with over 4 million on the waiting list in total. Without significant interventions through increased funding, capacity and staffing levels, the impact of Covid-19 is expected to last for many years, as can be seen by the fact that in 2023, waiting times for routine appointments are still at 18 weeks. Radical change to the delivery of routine care is to be expected in the coming years.

The government's handling of the pandemic

In general, the government's handling of the pandemic has drawn considerable criticism. In many cases, decisions about restrictions being put in place came much later than those in other countries with comparable infection figures, with the general perception being that needless deaths were caused by their belatedness. It was also felt by many that – as restrictions did ultimately result in bringing down case numbers, hospital admissions and the death toll – restrictions were lifted too soon and too dramatically, which ultimately led to further waves of infections.

Early on in the initial lockdown, it became apparent that there was not a sufficient amount of PPE for NHS and care workers, and millions of pounds were spent acquiring face masks that proved to be unusable. Advice was issued to frontline staff to wash and reuse PPE where necessary, which was regarded as a wholly inappropriate action. The general feeling was that NHS staff who were risking their own health and lives were being heavily let down.

There were also numerous occasions where members of the government breached lockdown rules, undermining public trust in their efforts to enforce national lockdown.

A positive and welcome response was the introduction of a number of economic support schemes, including the Furlough Scheme (where the government paid 80% of wages to those staff who were temporarily surplus to workplace requirements), which was ongoing until 30 September 2021, and the Self-Employed Income Support Scheme. These measures provided financial security to many in times of profound economic uncertainty.

In addition, the government provided funding for the development of Covid-19-specific Nightingale hospitals, and were also the first government to approve Covid-19 vaccinations.

At the time of writing, a public inquiry into the government's decision making during the pandemic was ongoing. At the end of its first phase, 69 scientists, civil servants, politicians and other experts had given their accounts of how prepared the healthcare system was ahead of the pandemic, and how well the UK had planned for it. So far, light has been shed on disagreements and tensions between the government and leading scientists. The inquiry, which should complete in 2024, hopes to identify lessons from which the government can learn, though they are not obliged to accept the recommendations in the final report.

Herd immunity

Early on in the pandemic, Sir Patrick Vallance, the government's chief scientific adviser, stated that transmission would be best reduced through the development of herd immunity. Herd immunity requires a large proportion of the population to become immune to an infectious agent, typically through a vaccination programme (see page 121). However, as the coronavirus responsible for Covid-19 was novel, there was no vaccine, and the government's early plans were to allow over 60% of the population to become infected with a virus with potentially devastating consequences. Understandably, this approach was heavily criticised, and the UK ultimately opted for a different approach.

Sweden was one country that adhered to the idea of natural herd immunity, without enforcing any national lockdowns, instead relying on voluntary social distancing, including working from home and avoiding public transport. In Sweden, other restrictions were also put in place, including banning large gatherings and restricted access to hospitality. The reasoning was that the restrictions would be long term and as such, this approach would be more manageable. Sweden's rates of infection remained comparable to other European countries that had more restrictive measures in place, without the devastating impact to Sweden's economy. However, while their approach was successful early on, death rates peaked in later months, with the Swedish population rapidly losing trust in their government's handling of the situation. Similarly, despite their approach, Sweden did not achieve herd immunity, with only 7% of the population possessing antibodies by the end of April 2021 – figures comparable to Spain and France, which both had prolonged lockdowns.

Vaccination programme

In general, the development of drugs and vaccines can take around 15 years on average for production and testing and is largely limited by funding and sufficient volunteers. The rapid spread of Covid-19 meant that the process was dramatically expedited through the provision of enormous funding awards and amendments to the way in which large-scale clinical trials were conducted in some countries, such as the US.

In addition, the mechanism that underpins two of the three widely used Covid-19 vaccines in the UK – produced by Moderna and Pfizer – also helped to speed up the process. Vaccines generally involve injection of an attenuated version of a pathogen, or recognisable elements of a pathogen, such as antigens (typically proteins on the surface of the pathogen). Both of these companies utilised the technology of mRNA vaccines – where a molecule of mRNA, or messenger RNA, that encodes a harmless version of a surface protein from the pathogen is injected, allowing the body to form its own version of the protein. This method avoids introducing a version of the virus to the vaccine recipient, does not affect their DNA in any way, and both the mRNA and protein break down quickly, making it very safe. While this is the first time an mRNA vaccine has been available to the public, research into mRNA vaccines for other diseases, such as flu, rabies and Zika virus has been underway for decades, making it a very well understood mechanism that will likely be used far more widely in the future.

The UK's contribution to the vaccination programme was the Oxford-AstraZeneca vaccine, which uses DNA rather than mRNA. They inserted the gene for the spike protein (discussed below) into a modified version of a chimpanzee-specific adenovirus, which typically cause illnesses like colds and flu. The virus can get inside the recipient's cells. While the virus itself is unable to replicate, the spike proteins can be synthesised by the host cells and they are presented on the surface of our own cells, so that our immune system can destroy them. In doing so, the immune system develops a memory of the spike protein so that upon infection by the Covid-19 virus, it is able to deal with it more readily.

For Covid-19 vaccines, the specific protein that was targeted was the spike protein, which covers the surface of all coronaviruses, which gives them a crown-like appearance when viewed under a microscope and therefore, their name. Viruses are particularly good at adapting to their environment, and undergo a process known as antigenic variation to alter their proteins through mutation. One potential cause for concern that was raised regarding the vaccines that were in use was that significant mutations in the spike protein could render the vaccine redundant as new strains emerged. In this sense, it is possible that the Covid-19 vaccine will follow the path of flu vaccines, where annual vaccinations are given to vulnerable individuals and those who choose to get them; these target strains that have emerged more recently.

While the mRNA vaccines were an incredible scientific breakthrough, they presented some logistical challenges, such as the need to store them at –80 degrees, making them difficult to transport quickly and safely and also difficult to store properly upon arrival. Given that the Oxford-AstraZeneca vaccine used DNA rather than mRNA – an infinitely more stable molecule – it could be stored at 4 degrees, which largely circumvented many of the issues that the mRNA vaccines presented.

The difficulties associated with accessibility and production of the vaccines, and the evident and unavoidable global demand, meant that there were immediate shortages. The vaccines were designed to be given as two doses, 21 days apart. However, the UK government opted to take an alternative approach. In order to immunise as many people as possible in the shortest time frame, they opted instead to give the second dose 12 weeks after the first, which deviated from the clinical trials that took place and prompted immediate questioning from some scientific experts regarding the efficacy of the vaccine if given in this way.

Despite these steps, the vaccination rollout was still slow in the UK initially. The first Pfizer-BioNTech vaccine was given in early December 2020, with hopes of vaccinating four million people by the end of the month. In reality, just 786,000 doses were given due to the problems outlined above. The approval of the Oxford-AstraZeneca vaccine for use from early January 2021 helped to alleviate some of these pressures, but did not eradicate them entirely.

Despite the relative success of the vaccination programme in the UK, vaccination in the UK generally has fallen in recent years, especially for the childhood vaccines, leading to a rise in the number of cases of diseases such as measles and mumps. While there are many potential reasons for this, much of the resistance to vaccination can be attributed to the continued spread of misinformation online. Anti-vaccination social media pages saw millions of new followers which led to discussions on the introduction of laws to prevent the spread of misinformation online.

Covid-19 gene

In November 2021, researchers at the University of Oxford identified a gene – LZTFL1 – that doubles the risk of respiratory failures in those that carry a certain version. The gene encodes a protein of the same name, abbreviated from leucine zipper transcription factor-like 1, which is thought to act as a tumour suppressor protein. Mutations have been associated with the development of malignant glioblastoma and benign schwannomatosis, which are cancers of the nervous system. As genes go, it is relatively unstudied, but it is likely that significant research will be conducted into its role in Covid-19 moving forward. The particular variant identified as problematic in Covid-19 is most commonly found in individuals of South Asian descent, which goes some way to explaining why some communities in the UK have been more significantly affected, as well as the impact that the virus has had in India. The research group responsible for its discovery have encouraged the communities most likely to carry the gene variant to get vaccinated and take precautions. It is likely that this is one of several genes that determine the impact of Covid-19, and more information will come to light with further research.

Treatment

As well as identification of a gene that causes significant problems following Covid-19 infection, November 2021 saw the UK approve the first oral drug to treat infected individuals in the UK. Molnupiravir inhibits one of the enzymes that the virus uses to replicate in host cells, meaning that the virus levels in the body should be kept low enough to prevent serious harm to vulnerable individuals in the population. As it can be administered in tablet form, it means that those who become unwell can take it at home, alleviating the pressure on hospitals by reducing the likelihood of admission. Initially, it is likely that its prescription will be restricted to those most at risk, such as older people with significant underlying health conditions, such as lung disease or cancer, though it is promising for the future.

Long Covid

Though the majority of people who are infected with Covid-19 make a recovery within weeks, others continue to experience symptoms for months to years. This condition is now being termed 'Long Covid', or 'post-Covid-19 syndrome'. As it is still a new condition that is being studied, it is largely undefined, but the most common symptoms include extreme fatigue, shortness of breath, aching muscles and loss of smell.

The NHS now has a Long Covid service, which is accessible through a GP referral, and is set up to provide additional support to aid recovery and manage symptoms. As more research into Long Covid is conducted, a better picture of the impacts of Covid-19 infection will emerge.

Things to consider

- In care homes mortality rates were extremely high due to the vulnerability of residents.
- Black, Asian and minority ethnic individuals were more affected by Covid-19 at its peak – this corresponded to black, Asian and minority ethnic workers making up a large proportion of key workers, but also leads to questions about institutional racism.
- The decline in the use of emergency care and how this has led to increased deaths in non-Covid-19 situations.
- The differing abilities of different regions to handle the demands of Covid-19 infections, due to differences in critical care facilities (i.e. intensive care beds were more available in London than other areas).
- The loss of primary care through GPs and its negative impact on the management of chronic conditions – with many appointments being online or over the phone, communication became inaccessible for some people, with important signs and symptoms being missed.
- The provision of mental health care declined and, where it remained, it predominantly moved to online or phone appointments, which prevented many people from making use of it due to a lack of privacy when confined to the family home.
- Economic and social impacts of lockdown and social distancing measures are likely to have enduring mental health effects.
- The effectiveness of restrictions such as lockdowns and social distancing for those living in more socially and economically deprived areas, especially with lower incomes and overcrowding, which highlights significant health inequalities in the UK.
- The weaknesses of the NHS that were highlighted by the pandemic – a lack of funding, staffing shortfall and lack of specialist equipment.
- As well as disparities between regions of the UK, different countries around the world were impacted differently, with those with greater economic stability (and related benefits such as better nutrition and housing conditions) and solid borders faring better.
- Sweden's response: it did not enforce a national lockdown yet did not observe the consequences anticipated by the UK.
- The spread of misinformation by anti-vaxxers online gaining traction and potentially hampering the vaccination programme.
- The continued advances in scientific technology allowing for the production of successful vaccines and drugs, as well as the identification of genes that increase the risk of death.
- Long Covid is still a relatively new and unstudied condition that is affecting a proportion of those who get infected by Covid-19.

Useful websites

- NHS: www.nhs.uk/conditions/coronavirus-covid-19
- World Health Organization: www.who.int/emergencies/diseases/novel-coronavirus-2019
- Statista: www.statista.com/topics/5994/the-coronavirus-disease-covid-19-outbreak
- BBC: www.bbc.co.uk/news/coronavirus

When reading about the pandemic in the media, consider investigating different news sources to ensure that your understanding is unbiased.

Cervical cancer

With 3,200 new cases each year, cervical cancer is the 14th most common cancer in the UK. It can affect anyone with a cervix, and is most common in those aged below 45. Cervical cancer is unusual in that the majority of cases are caused by infection with a virus, known as the human papillomavirus (HPV), which is sexually transmitted. For the most part, HPV does not cause any problems in those that carry it, though in a small proportion of people, it can remain in the cells of the cervix and ultimately lead to the development of cancer. Being a virus, it was possible to produce a vaccine against HPV and, in turn, cervical cancer. The vaccine programme has been in place since 2006, with teenagers receiving the vaccine from the age of 12, with a view to the immune system developing protection against HPV prior to sexual activity.

In 2023, it was reported that between 80–90% of UK teenagers receive the vaccine, which is thought to be 90% effective against HPV transmission. As with any vaccination programme, once successfully established, it is hoped that disease eradication could be possible. Vaccination, however, is only part of the reason why cervical cancer could be the first cancer to be eradicated; it is also heavily reliant on cervical screening for pre-cancerous cells. The NHS provides a cervical screening service to women aged between 25 and 64, where pre-emptive measures can be put in place ahead of cervical cancer developing.

The WHO had outlined plans to eradicate cervical cancer by the end of the century, but in November 2023, NHS England boss Amanda Pritchard stated that the UK is on track to eliminate cervical cancer by 2040, owing to the recent increase in the uptake of the HPV vaccination. On the other hand, recent statistics suggest that the number of people attending cervical screening appointments is declining, though it is possible that the most recent data are impacted by the Covid-19 pandemic. Providing both vaccination and cervical screening attendance rates continue to increase, the eradication of cervical cancer – and the first possibility of eradicating any type of cancer – may be in sight.

Sickle cell anaemia and Beta-thalassemia

Many diseases and conditions around the world are caused by known variations in individual genes. In recent years, modern technologies have developed that have allowed for genetic manipulation and have been commonly used as research tools, with a view to ultimately using them as a means of treating, or at least managing, genetic conditions – this is known as gene therapy. In November 2023, the UK Medicines and Healthcare Products Regulatory Agency approved the first gene therapy drug, specifically to cure sickle-cell disease and transfusion-dependent Beta-thalassemia.

Gene therapy is a technique that can be used to modify the genome of specific cells, with a view to treating or preventing the development of genetic conditions. Casgevy, the approved drug, works on the principles of gene therapy by using a gene-editing tool known as CRISPR. Put simply, the CRISPR system can be viewed as a pair of 'molecular scissors'. Guide RNA, or gRNA, is designed to be complementary to the affected region of the gene of interest. The gRNA is combined with an enzyme called Cas9, and guides the enzyme to the affected DNA. Theer, the enzyme functions as the molecular scissors by making a cut in the DNA to prevent it producing the faulty, disease-causing protein. Though this is a very oversimplified description of the technology, it is clear that many diseases could be treated, or at least controlled, in this manner. In the case of Casgevy, patients' haematopoietic stem cells are removed from the bone marrow and edited in a laboratory. Their remaining stem cells must be destroyed through chemotherapy and/or radiotherapy – a trade-off that clinical trial patients largely felt outweighed the potential risks – before the genetically modified cells are infused back into the patient.

Sickle cell anaemia and Beta-thalassemia are ideal targets of a CRISPR-based therapy due to both of the inherited blood disorders being caused by mutations in a single gene, specifically the Beta-globin gene. This gene is responsible for the production of the Beta-globin chain in haemoglobin, which is the protein responsible for transporting oxygen around the body. In sickle cell disease, the resulting fault in the protein changes the overall haemoglobin structure to the point that red blood cells become 'sickle shaped' and thus are less efficient at transporting oxygen; these cells can also block the narrowest blood vessels, causing extreme pain and increasing the risk of cardiac events, such as heart attacks and strokes. Beta-thalassemia is also caused by a range of mutations in this gene, with the outcome being a lack of functional haemoglobin in circulation. Patients of both diseases require lifelong treatments and condition management, with no existing cure.

As diseases that have largely been neglected in terms of advancing treatments and finding cures, approval of Casgevy is a huge step, especially as a one-off treatment should be sufficient to be curative. However, as it is a personalised treatment that is specific to each individual patient, with their own cells being modified on a case by case basis, it is likely to be expensive and time-consuming, and as such, extremely limited in its availability.

Strep A

In December 2022, concerns over the common bacteria strep A hit the media after several children in the UK died from related infection. While many people carry a non-infectious form of strep A in their bodies, mutant forms of the bacteria can cause illness, such as a sore throat or skin infection, though these are typically mild and readily treated. Strep A infections are contracted through coughs and sneezes, as well as close contact. As such, areas where people are closely confined, such as schools, are more likely to see such outbreaks. Strep A can also cause scarlet fever, which is common in young children, and is characterised by flu-like symptoms, a rash that feels like sandpaper, and a 'strawberry tongue'.

On rare occasions, strep A can cause invasive group A streptococcal infection (iGAS), which can be fatal. Generally, this occurs when the bacteria enter the blood stream. It is most common in those with weaker immune systems, such as immunocompromised people, the elderly and young children. While this led to a number of deaths and many severe illnesses in young children in the UK in winter 2022, there is no evidence to suggest that a new strain of strep A was the cause; rather it is being attributed to a larger number of bacteria in circulation that were being transmitted more readily in the absence of Covid restrictions.

Both iGAS and scarlet fever are notifiable diseases, meaning that local health protection teams must be alerted to diagnosed cases so that mechanisms can be put in place to manage outbreaks and reduce further transmission. Between 7 November and 11 December 2022, 9,945 cases of scarlet fever were reported, which was a significant increase. Also higher than normal were iGAS notifications, with 509 in the same time period, showing a similar but less pronounced rise, presumably as a consequence of the increased scarlet fever diagnoses.

Brexit

The NHS became a political battleground once again in 2016 as the Brexit vote loomed large. The Brexit campaign will be synonymous with the image of Boris Johnson on his battle bus, with the slogan, 'We send £350 million a week to the EU. Let's fund our NHS instead.' However, the slogan, like the promise, has transpired to be misleading, and the £350 million promised during the EU referendum has not materialised. Some additional funding was promised in 2019: the government pledged an increase of £33.9 billion to the NHS budget by 2024. In recent years, additional funding has been provided for Covid-19, to help deal with the vast increase in hospital admissions.

Since the UK formally left the EU in 2020, some potential areas of concern have come to light, though the extent of these may not yet have been fully realised. So, what impact has Brexit had on the NHS so far, and what other issues might come to light?

- New customs checks at the border and paperwork have meant delays and complications, at least initially.
- A shortage of lorry drivers caused problems in September 2021, which impacted the import of medicines into the UK.
- An end to mutual recognition of professional qualifications, although the UK has decided to continue to recognise EEA qualifications for up to two years, but there is no reciprocity. This could further impact on the NHS's current staffing problems.
- EU/EEA students are now classed as international students for fee purposes and no longer benefit from Home student fees and financial support. This may deter outstanding students in medicine, nursing and other related healthcare fields from studying and working in the UK.

In a 2022 report from the Nuffield Trust, it became apparent that concerns regarding staffing numbers were justified, with a loss of over 10,000 healthcare staff from the EU. Recruitment of staff from the rest of the world has increased to make up some of the shortfall, but, overall, this is insufficient to recover the entire workforce. Some particular areas, such as cardiothoracic surgery and anaesthetics, have been hit particularly hard. These shortages then impact remaining staff by increasing pressure and reducing morale due to enhanced workloads. Ethically, recruiting healthcare staff from countries experiencing their own structural workforce issues is highly problematic. The new points-based immigration system for people wanting to come and work in the UK is unlikely to exclude most healthcare workers (although care workers will be adversely affected).

In addition, drug shortages have meant that pharmacists have been permitted to use waivers that allow them to pay higher prices, increasing the financial demands on the NHS.

Fortunately, in September 2023, the Prime Minister secured a deal that allowed UK scientists to benefit from the EU's scientific research and innovation programme, Horizon Europe, with certainty until 2027, by being permitted to make applications for funding.

Black, Asian and minority ethnic communities

The Covid-19 pandemic brought to light a startling statistic – the mortality and morbidity of the virus was heavily skewed towards black, Asian and minority ethnic groups (BAME) among both staff and patients. The NHS recognised this as 'not just an equality, diversity and inclusion issue' but an 'urgent medical emergency' that required immediate action. In May 2020, the Chief Medical Officer asked Public Health England to explore the impact of Covid-19 across different population groups through analysis of various factors, such as confirmed cases, hospitalisations and deaths by ethnicity. They focussed on several key areas.

- Protection of staff through thorough risk assessments, with an emphasis on the mental and physical health of BAME staff.
- Increased engagement with BAME staff to learn from lived experience.
- BAME representation in decision-making processes.
- Emphasis on the rehabilitation and recovery of BAME staff through ongoing support to meet emotional needs.

While Covid-19 may have brought these issues to the fore, they have been deep-rooted for a long time. Very few board members are from BAME backgrounds, and a lack of diversity at senior levels has resulted in white applicants being 1.46 times more likely to be appointed than their BAME peers. To overcome this, institutional racism and unconscious bias need to be addressed, and the NHS has set out to achieve this through the steps outlined above, but predominantly through increased BAME representation at all levels in the workforce and increased reflection on the experiences of BAME communities to learn from their experiences.

'Our Future Health'

In October 2022, the NHS rolled out its 'Our Future Health' programme. This will be the UK's largest ever health research programme, which aims to identify disease in patients prior to the onset of symptoms. The goal is 'to transform the prevention, detection and treatment of conditions such as dementia, cancer, diabetes, heart disease and stroke', to enable better health across the whole population.

The programme will work by taking blood samples and physical health measurements from volunteers across the UK. By doing so, it will aim to identify biomarkers and causative factors that contribute to disease that have a symptomatic onset later in life. At the time of writing, it is in its very early stages, but research programmes such as this are set to transform the clinical landscape in the UK. Throughout the later months of 2023, many new clinics opened across the UK to enhance the recruitment of volunteers.

Apps and virtual technology in medicine

It is a brave new world, and there is an increasing trend now for the use of apps and virtual technology in order to help patients. The latest innovation is being able to get an appointment with a GP; Push Doctor and Now GP are the two leading services to do this, reportedly being able to reach over 1 million patients. This reduces waiting times and gains quicker access to doctors. Only the future will show whether this will prove as effective as seeing a GP in person.

This concept has also extended into hospitals, where a Virtual Fracture Clinic is in operation at hospitals such as the Brighton and Sussex group of hospitals in order to assess more minor injuries over the phone and then refer the patient to the virtual fracture clinic for physiotherapy exercises and monitoring, thus reducing the waiting lists of those waiting for hospital appointments.

Mental health

Owing to an increased awareness of mental health conditions, they are being diagnosed more frequently, and account for a significant proportion of the total burden of disease. In 2021, 5,583 suicides were registered in England and Wales, with men being three times more likely to take their own lives than women in the UK. As these numbers continue to rise, there has been a multitude of mental health campaigns, by both charities and Public Health England. Irrespective of how successful these campaigns are in encouraging people to seek the help that they need, the support is not always freely available through the NHS.

There is no parity between provisions for the treatment of mental and physical health conditions; just 14% of the NHS's budget is given to mental health care. Despite mental health issues being a growing concern, NHS mental health services have been reduced in a number of regions. As such, those suffering with mental health conditions, especially young people, are being failed by the NHS due to long waiting lists or a complete absence of available options.

According to the Mental Health Foundation, the most commonly diagnosed mental health problems are:

- anxiety
- depression
- bipolar disorder
- schizophrenia
- stress.

CCGs have been called into question regarding their funding allocations for mental health provisions. At present, the NHS is rolling out significant changes that should ultimately improve the landscape.

- An increase in the provision of psychological therapies, such as cognitive behavioural therapy.
- The development of digital therapies, which can be accessed rapidly.
- Improved support for high-risk groups including children and young people and pregnant or new mothers.
- Reducing the travel requirements by increasing care availability closer to home.
- The introduction of specialist mental health care in A&E departments.
- More thorough physical health checks for mental health patients.
- The introduction of specialist mental health services for veterans.

In recent years, there has been a huge movement around the theme of mindfulness, which is a way of managing thought processes and feelings and, ultimately, mental health. Mindfulness exercises allow an individual to focus on the present moment, and are a recommended treatment for those with mental health conditions. There are numerous approaches, including yoga, meditation and breathing techniques. The Mental Health Foundation, in partnership with Be Mindful, has produced an online course in mindfulness.

NHS England is currently running a campaign called Every Mind Matters, which outlines the things that individuals can do to help manage their own mental health, as well as pointing people in the direction of information about different mental health issues, and where to get support. It also promotes the production of an 'action plan', which involves taking minor actions to improve mental health, such as:

- being more active
- undertaking social interaction
- reframing unhelpful thoughts
- being mindful, or in the present
- developing good sleep habits
- being in control of your day
- minimising worries
- carrying out self-care
- getting help and support where required.

The Covid-19 pandemic and its associated lockdowns have undoubtedly had a negative impact on the mental health of the global population. Recent studies highlighted a decline in the mental health of the UK population when compared to trends pre-pandemic, with women, young people and those with very young children being the most affected.

Things to consider

- The burden of mental health conditions on the NHS should not be underestimated.
- Mental health problems can be associated with a number of physical health problems.
- Either in conjunction with their associated physical health problems or independently, mental health problems contribute enormously to absenteeism.
- An individual's mental health is as important as their physical health, and NHS provisions should reflect this.

TIP!

NHS England runs a number of campaigns to address wider healthcare issues. It is worth keeping up to date with current campaigns, either by taking note of advertisements or looking at their website.

Vaccinations

A large focus of the NHS is preventative medicine. One of the ways in which the spread of disease can be minimised is through the use of vaccination. The basis of vaccination is that by introducing a weakened form of the pathogen into the body of an individual, their immune system will generate a full-blown response. In the case of infection by the live pathogen, the immune system will be in place to prevent the development of disease. As such, vaccines can present a straightforward way of minimising the spread of preventable disease. Time and money are put into vaccination programmes for a number of reasons.

- Vaccines prevent infection with diseases that can be fatal, thereby providing a successful means of saving lives.
- All vaccines are thoroughly tested for safety before being used on a large scale.
- They are regarded as being completely safe for widespread use.
- Adverse reactions, such as allergies, are possible but incredibly rare.
- Vaccination programmes allow for 'herd immunity'; by vaccinating the majority of a vulnerable population, the pathogen responsible for causing disease will have difficulty spreading from person to person.
- Vaccines can protect future generations, as a vaccinated mother cannot pass an infection on to her unborn child.
- Successful vaccination programmes can eradicate disease, as was the case with smallpox.
- Vaccines are more cost-effective than the treatment and management of disease caused by the infection that is being prevented.

Despite strong scientific evidence suggesting that, for the most part, vaccines are safe and effective, there has been a large movement in recent years of 'anti-vaxxers', who completely disagree with the notion of vaccination, citing numerous reasons.

- Vaccines can cause serious and, in some cases, fatal side effects.
- Vaccines can contain potentially harmful chemical compounds, such as heavy metal traces, or ingredients that some individuals see as being immoral, such as animal products.
- Vaccines cannot be mandatory, as this infringes upon human rights.
- Natural immunity is more robust than vaccines, which are unnatural.
- Vaccines target diseases which, owing to previously successful vaccination programmes, have been almost eradicated.
- In some cases, the diseases that the vaccines protect against are relatively harmless, and carry less risk than the vaccine.

One of the major contributors to the anti-vaxxer movement was the controversy associated with the combined measles, mumps and rubella (MMR) vaccine. Each infection is highly contagious and can lead to significant complications, such as deafness, encephalitis and meningitis, as well as miscarriage in pregnancy. The side effects of the MMR vaccine were mild compared to vaccinating for each disease independently, and, after its introduction in 1988, the number of cases of each disease dropped considerably.

However, in 1998, Dr Andrew Wakefield published a study in the respected and peer-reviewed medical journal *The Lancet*, linking the MMR vaccine to the development of autism in children. The media response to this caused a retreat by many from the vaccination programme, and a subsequent increase in measles, mumps and rubella. Since the publication, it was found that Dr Wakefield had fabricated the results and his work has been entirely discredited. Subsequent studies conducted on a much larger scale have found no link between the MMR jab and autism. Despite this, many people still believe that there is a link.

In November 2018, Professor Dame Sally Davies, the former chief medical officer for England, encouraged parents to ignore the myths spread on social media by anti-vaccine campaigners, branding them as 'fake news'. The number of individuals vaccinated currently sits at 87%, which falls significantly short of the 95% required for herd immunity.

In December 2020, the first vaccinations against Covid-19 were introduced. The vaccine rollout has been largely successful in protecting the majority of the population from severe Covid-19 infections, but there has been a significant anti-vaxxer movement. The vaccine for the pandemic is discussed in more detail in the Covid-19 section above.

Things to consider

Typically, people have a specific opinion and are either fully for or against vaccination. For medical school interviews, it is worth researching these points in greater depth so that you can confidently talk through both sides of the argument. It is worth remembering that it is the right of the parent or guardian to decide whether or not children are vaccinated.

Dementia

Dementia is a collective term for a group of brain disorders that result in a progressive loss of brain function. Among the diseases described by dementia, Alzheimer's disease is the most common, with between 50% and 75% of diagnosed individuals affected by it. Over the last few years, the term 'dementia' has been used far more frequently by the media, and this can be attributed to the vast increase in the number of diagnosed cases and resulting deaths.

Different forms of dementia

There are numerous different forms of dementia, including:

- Alzheimer's disease
- vascular dementia
- dementia with Lewy bodies
- frontotemporal dementia.

It can also arise from more rare conditions, such as:

- Huntington's disease
- corticobasal degeneration
- progressive supranuclear palsy
- normal pressure hydrocephalus.

You are not expected to have a great deal of understanding about the biological basis of dementia in each of these diseases, but it is worth considering that the progression of each disease differs significantly, making it harder to diagnose and treat each individual.

Why are the numbers increasing so drastically?

In 2018, dementia and Alzheimer's disease were once again the leading cause of death in the UK according to the Office for National Statistics, accounting for 12.7% of recorded deaths. There are thought to be around 850,000 people living with a form of dementia in the UK, with

In the news - link to football

For several years, the link between heading the ball in football and dementia has been explored. In 2018, researchers identified the condition 'chronic traumatic encephalopathy' (CTE), and pushed for heading the ball, even at a professional level, to be restricted. Much of the momentum surrounding this research came following the death of former professional footballer Jeff Astle as a result of brain trauma from heading the older, and considerably heavier, leather footballs.

In July 2021, the Football Association (FA) released guidance on heading the ball at both a professional and amateur level. Initially, this guidance focuses on heading the ball in training sessions, where it occurs most frequently, and on headers that have a higher force. It is recommended that headers that are of a higher force be limited to ten per week in training, with clubs considering other factors – such as how many headers a player is likely to be involved in per game, the position they play in, their age and their gender. For specific heading practice sessions, throwing the ball is recommended rather than kicking, to ensure that force is lower.

For the 2022–2023 season, the FA initiated a trial that looked at the impact of not heading the ball in U12 (under 12-year-olds) football. The trial has been extended for the 2023–2024 season, with a view that from 2024–2025, heading the ball could be banned entirely for this age category.

the number of cases expected to exceed 1.5 million by 2040. Reasons for this include the following.

- An ageing population – individuals now have a longer life expectancy, and dementia is more common in elderly people.
- Better healthcare provisions for other leading causes of death – cardiovascular disease, among other leading causes of death, can now be treated and managed more effectively, which is reducing the death toll for these diseases.
- Greater awareness – dementia is now being cited as a cause of death more frequently owing to an improved understanding of the disease by healthcare professionals.

At present, there is no cure for the different forms of dementia. A huge focus of healthcare professionals at the moment is prevention of the disease, or at least delaying the onset in those at high risk.

Some of the risk factors for dementia include:

- age – dementia is more likely to develop in older age
- genetic predisposition – there are a number of gene variants that are thought to be linked with the onset of dementia.

New research has also linked the following to the onset of dementia:

- lower levels of education
- hearing loss
- untreated depression
- social isolation
- sedentary lifestyles.

Lifestyle medicine, a term used with a much higher frequency of late, is being branded as a means of reducing the risk of developing a number of diseases, including those encompassed by dementia. The logic is that a healthy lifestyle, as reflected by a balanced diet (which is high in fibre, and low in saturated fat, salt and sugar), maintaining a healthy weight, regular exercise, stopping smoking and minimising alcohol intake, is likely to prevent disease from occurring. By the time that diagnosis has occurred, the damage to the brain is too significant to reverse, which is why the focus is on early intervention.

Air pollution

Air pollution is classified as the introduction of harmful or excessive quantities of substances into the Earth's atmosphere, such as gases, particulate matter and biological molecules. Breathing is absolutely vital to staying alive, but walking along a busy city street makes that crucial act incredibly risky. With 99% of the world's population living in an area where air pollution levels do not meet World Health Organization air quality guidelines, it's no wonder that the health implications are becoming an increasing concern. The statistics show that most countries are at risk of the consequences of air pollution, but the most significant burden is in low- and middle-income countries.

What are the pollutants?

- Particulate matter
- Ozone
- Nitrogen dioxide
- Sulphur dioxide

On average, 4.2 million deaths worldwide are attributed to ambient air pollution each year. These are predominantly a result of:

- lung cancer
- respiratory infections
- stroke
- heart disease
- chronic obstructive pulmonary disease (COPD).

Both child and adult health can be impaired by air pollution, whether it is either short- or long-term. Most commonly, it is associated with compromised lung function, more frequent respiratory infections and aggravation of conditions such as asthma. In addition, exposure to air pollution in expectant mothers is thought to lead to adverse outcomes at birth.

In the UK, the Department for Environment, Food and Rural Affairs provides guidelines to minimise the impact of air pollution at peak times, especially in high-risk groups. Some examples include:

- reducing levels of outdoor exercise when pollution levels are high
- limited exertion on high pollution days by the elderly and those with heart and lung conditions
- continuing the use of medication as advised by healthcare practitioners for asthmatics, and increasing the use of inhaled reliever medication where required.

The department's advice is summarised in Table 6 overleaf.

The World Health Organization published a roadmap in 2016, outlining key areas that it planned to address in the near future.

- Improving public knowledge of the impacts of air pollution on health.
- Improving the reporting on health trends associated with air pollution.
- Improved utilisation of the healthcare sector to meet the above targets locally, nationally, regionally and globally.

In addition, a number of Sustainable Development Goals have been put in place. Essentially, these are a list of targets put in place to improve global health in relation to air pollution.

- A significant decrease in the reduction of air pollution-related deaths and illnesses.
- Access to clean energy in homes to reduce the output of air pollution.
- Access to sustainable, safe and affordable transport methods.
- Reducing the environmental impact of cities.

It is worth researching what is being done in your city to meet these goals. In the UK, several cities, including Bath, Birmingham, Bradford, Bristol, Portsmouth, Sheffield and Tyneside have clean air zones in place, with plans for Greater Manchester currently under review. The idea is that polluting vehicles must pay to use major roads to enter the city centre, with a view to deterring people from using vehicles that do not meet specific pollution standards and to encourage them to make use of public transport instead. The reliance on individual local authorities to take action has been viewed as insufficient however, and companies such as ClientEarth have repeatedly taken the UK government to court regarding these inadequacies.

Irrespective of the effectiveness of these interventions, there is no doubt that the developed world is trying to improve this situation owing to an improved understanding of its impact on health. As promising as this is, the developing world is getting worse, and air pollution is now regarded as a public health emergency.

Table 6 DEFRA guidelines

Air Pollution banding	Value	Accompanying health messages for at-risk groups and the general populace	
		At-risk individuals	General population
Low	1–3	**Enjoy** your usual outdoor activities.	**Enjoy** your usual outdoor activities.
Moderate	4–6	Adults and children with lung problems, and adults with heart problems, **who experience symptoms**, should **consider reducing** strenuous physical activity, particularly outdoors.	**Enjoy** your usual outdoor activities.
High	7–9	Adults and children with lung problems, and adults with heart problems, should **reduce** strenuous physical exertion, particularly if they experience symptoms. People with asthma may find they need to use their reliever inhaler more often. Older people should **reduce** physical exertion.	Anyone experiencing discomfort such as sore eyes, cough or sore throat should **consider reducing** activity, particularly outdoors.
Very high	10	Adults and children with lung problems, adults with heart problems, and older people, should **avoid** strenuous physical exertion. People with asthma may find they need to use their reliever inhaler more often.	**Reduce** physical exertion, particularly outdoors, especially if you experience symptoms such as cough or sore throat.

Source: https://uk-air.defra.gov.uk/air-pollution/daqi?view=effects.

Case study

In February 2013, nine-year-old Ella Kissi-Debrah tragically passed away from a fatal asthma attack. Ella lived in close proximity to one of London's busiest roads, and had been hospitalised 27 times in the three years preceding her death. In 2019, a new inquest into Ella's death was initiated to investigate whether unlawful levels of air pollution were a contributing factor. In a landmark case, the coroner concluded that Ella died from acute respiratory failure, asthma and 'air pollution exposure'. This is the first time that air pollution has been declared as a contributory cause of illness and death.

Personalised medicine

The current approach to medicine is, for the most part, 'one size fits all': once a patient is diagnosed with a condition, they might be given a drug or a treatment programme that is generic to that particular disease. However, with most conditions, there are individual cases where the method of treatment is ineffective and, for a long time, this was put down to individual differences that could not be helped.

One such example is the treatment of heart disease (or more specifically, coronary artery disease) by a drug known as clopidogrel, which prevents the formation of blood clots. In 2010, clopidogrel was the second most widely prescribed drug in the USA, despite reports of marked variability between patient responses. In short, doctors were aware that the drug might not be effective, but as it was still the most effective treatment available, they prescribed it anyway.

Fast forward several years and countless studies later, and scientists have pinpointed the reason for its outstanding effectiveness in some patients and the complete lack of impact in others. The drug works by targeting a specific enzyme in the liver, but due to genetic differences between individuals, the structure of these enzymes can differ significantly. If a patient does not have the specific enzyme that clopidogrel acts upon, it will not work, and they are still at an extremely high risk of having a heart attack.

Understanding the mechanism of action of the drug and the varied responses was incredibly important, but it led to a bigger question: what can be done about this clinically? A genetic test emerged and was used by some private healthcare companies in the USA that, in a couple of hours, allowed doctors to see whether or not the drug would be effective. For numerous reasons, such as the tests available being in their early stages and a lack of large-scale studies and clinical trials, these specific tests have not been rolled out nationally or globally just yet. However, it nicely outlines the basis of precision medicine.

Precision medicine is a movement that is working towards the better management of patient health by ascertaining individual differences and using therapies that are targeted to them directly. Ultimately, this should result in improved health outcomes and an overall reduced cost of healthcare owing to the improved specificity of the treatments provided.

The concept of personalised medicine has been around for a long time, but advances in technology are allowing for the identification of useful interventions, and even whether an individual is at risk of developing a particular disease. The NHS has outlined the advantages of personalised medicine as 'the four Ps'.

The four Ps of personalised medicine

1. **Prediction and prevention of disease.** New technologies will allow for the identification of diagnostic markers that indicate an individual is likely to develop a particular disease, even before they show symptoms. This could allow for advice to be given on adopting better lifestyle choices, and provide an opportunity for early treatment.
2. **Precise diagnosis.** Two patients diagnosed with the same disease as they have the same symptoms may not necessarily mean that the cause of their disease is the same. As such, personalised medicine will allow for each individual's molecular and cellular processes to be carefully analysed, so that the specific nature of their disease can be understood.
3. **Personalised interventions.** As the origin of the disease can be identified, treatment methods can also be provided in a very specific manner. This could be through the prescription of a specific drug, or even a point-of-care genetic test to establish what the best treatment option might be. In doing so, the NHS will be able to move away from the 'trial and error' approach to treating disease, which is costly and can result in adverse drug responses.
4. **Participation of patients.** By improving understanding, doctors can talk to patients about what they can do to help themselves. In many diseases, improving lifestyle factors can prevent the onset of a disease that they are predisposed to, or help with the management of a disease with which they have already been diagnosed.

In light of the enormous funding pressures on the NHS, the introduction of personalised medicine could assist with the alleviation of resource allocation issues. While the integration of technologies may be costly initially, in the long term, the costs of diagnosis and treatment will be much reduced, as less money will be wasted on inefficient treatments and unnecessary diagnostic tests.

The science of genomics

The movement of genomics – a term relating to the science of genetics, but using advanced technology – has really paved the way for personalised medicine and underpins every aspect of it.

The Human Genome Project, completed in 2003, was an enormous undertaking that involved the collective efforts of scientists globally over a 15-year period and, at the time, cost an extortionate $3 billion. Nowadays, a whole human genome can be sequenced in a matter of hours for less than £1000, and these prices continue to fall. It is these technological advances that have made the possibility of sequencing each individual genome a reality.

The sequencing of whole genomes is referred to as Whole Genome Sequencing (WGS), and there are many institutions worldwide that have conducted large scale projects. In the UK alone there are many significant projects, but the one that has had the largest impact to date is the 100,000 Genomes Project.

The 100,000 Genomes Project

The 100,000 Genomes Project was initiated by former Prime Minister David Cameron, who allocated funding to the project in 2012 for the sequencing of 100,000 genomes of NHS patients and their relatives who were affected by rare and poorly understood genetic diseases and cancers. The initial aims of the project were to identify the causes of rare diseases and allow new medical research to take place to identify treatments and cures for what are typically fatal and devastating conditions. The 100,000th sequence was achieved in December 2018. Now, the project aims to support the NHS with improved treatment of conditions as it moves towards an era of personalised medicine.

Despite the enormous promise that projects such as the 100,000 Genomes Project and the notion of personalised medicine present, there are some reservations.

- Genomics is an enormous data science – that is to say, vast quantities of personal data, in the form of genomes, are being stored and obtained for free. There are concerns about the safety of that data, or even that there may be commercial gain for companies from information that has been provided by patients for free.
- Ethical concerns – some issues have been raised about the knowledge of the state of a patient's health. Some concerns have been raised over whether or not patients should be given information about additional potential health problems revealed by their genome (for example, if a doctor is looking to establish which treatment is best for a heart condition, and discovers that the patient is also likely to develop a particular form of cancer).

In July 2018, headlines stated that a new, routine DNA test will put the NHS at the forefront of medicine. The tests referred to in the headline are routine genomic tests for individuals diagnosed with cancer that will allow for the reading, analysis and interpretation of tumour DNA by specialist genomics centres around the UK. In doing so, the specific molecular cause of the cancer can be identified, and patients can be 'matched' with the most effective treatment, minimising adverse responses to drugs in the process. These new tests were rolled out across the UK on 1 October 2018, and look to be the first tangible step in the NHS's move towards personalised medicine.

In 2022, the NHS set out its accelerating genomic medicine strategy to embed genomics into routine care over the next five years. This will result in the NHS being able to deliver tailored treatment and reduce adverse drug reactions, leading to improved outcomes for patients with cancer and genetic diseases. In addition, it will allow genomic data to be used alongside and to inform other clinical data for more robust diagnostics and treatment plans. A summary of the integration of genomics into the NHS and what it means can be found at www.england.nhs.uk/long-read/genomics.

Ageing population

Globally, life expectancy continues to rise (except in many sub-Saharan African countries, which have been ravaged by HIV/AIDS) because of improvements in sanitation and medical care. According to the WHO, the number of people aged 60 or over will increase to 2.1 billion by 2050, from 1 billion in 2019. Birth rates in most countries are falling, and the combination of the two brings considerable problems. The relative number of people who succumb to chronic illness (such as cancer, diabetes or diseases of the circulatory system) is increasing, and this puts greater strain on countries' healthcare systems.

It is a well-reported fact that the population of the UK is ageing. The Office for National Statistics (ONS) reports that 18.6% of the UK population were aged over 65 in 2021, and this is expected to rise. These statistics can be attributed to the continuing developments in technology, improvements in healthcare and a better quality of lifestyle, all of which are contributing to people living longer lives.

Perhaps the most important aspects to consider are the challenges that an ageing population presents. Predominantly, these challenges come in the form of increased healthcare demands, and an associated increase in healthcare costs. This is attributable to an increase in the diagnosis of diseases that are more common in elderly people, such as dementia.

As technology and healthcare continue to improve, it is unlikely that life expectancy will fall. As such, there is a new focus by the NHS in partnership with Age UK to change the view of old age: rather than reacting to the frailty of the elderly, we must now start to take a proactive approach to reducing it.

Things to consider

It is worth considering some of the differences in life expectancy in different populations when preparing for interviews, as these differences may point you in the direction of mechanisms put in place by different healthcare systems.

- Why does Japan have the highest life expectancy?
- Why does France have a higher life expectancy than the UK?
- Why are most of the countries with the lowest Health Adjusted Life Expectancy (HALE) figures located in the middle and southern parts of Africa?

You can probably guess the answers to these, but, if not, further data is available at www.who.int/gho/en.

Lifestyle factors

Obesity

Obesity is an increasing problem throughout the UK, especially in the younger generation. With the UK at the top of the European obesity league, it is a big issue and very much an interview question. The last recorded Health Survey for England of 2021 (published in 2022) revealed that 26% of adults are clinically obese and 69% of men and 59% of women are overweight or obese. Obesity is defined as having a body mass index (BMI) of above 30. The annual cost to the NHS in 2023 was roughly £6.2 billion (estimated to be £9.7 billion by 2050), and £49.9 billion to the wider economy.

The main causes of obesity are a combination of a lack of exercise and the consumption of excessive calories. Obesity has detrimental effects on many components of the human body, especially in later life. The extra body weight means the heart has to work harder and therefore there is an increase in blood pressure: this can lead to coronary heart disease. Atherosclerosis often occurs, which is a build-up of cholesterol and fatty substances in the lining of the arteries; this reduces the flow of blood, and therefore oxygen, to the heart muscle or other tissues such as the brain. Without oxygen, even for a short time, cells in these tissues die. Obesity has also been shown, among other conditions, to cause respiratory problems, type 2 diabetes, and osteoarthritis due to the strain on the joints.

As a consequence of the numerous lockdowns and restricted activity due to the Covid-19 pandemic, it is predicted that the UK's obesity statistics will worsen in the coming years. Although obesity in the UK has been a longstanding problem, Covid-19 brought it back into focus because those that were obese were at greater risk of being admitted to hospital, of being admitted to intensive care units and, ultimately, of dying. Public Health England and the government released a call to action for the UK population to move towards a healthier weight. The campaign involved the release of new apps to help people manage their weight, banning advertisements for foods that are high in fats, sugars and salt before 9pm online and on TV, introducing legislation to restrict volume promotions of these foods (e.g. buy one get one free), and introducing calorie labels to food and alcohol more widely.

Childhood obesity

According to the government's Health Survey for England, in 2019, 1.6 million children aged 2 to 15 years were estimated to be obese. It is a fact that children with obese parents are more likely to be obese than children with healthier parents, and almost twice as many children living in the most deprived areas were obese as those living in the least deprived areas. It is reported that a quarter of children aged 2 to 15 years spend at least six hours every weekend day being inactive. This is the highest rate in Western Europe and contributes to the estimated overall annual cost of obesity of approximately £6 billion to the NHS in the UK. In order to address the dangers that obesity can have for children's health, the Chartered Society of Physiotherapy has published extensive guidelines designed to try and engage parents and young children with the idea of regular exercise in a healthy lifestyle. In light of these statistics, it is clear that this issue is immensely important in terms of both preventing our children from becoming obese as well as protecting future generations.

Why is obesity a problem?

Obesity is linked to a number of health problems, including:

- coronary heart disease (CHD)
- type 2 diabetes
- increased risk of a number of cancers
- stroke
- high blood pressure
- high cholesterol levels
- asthma
- gallstones
- sleep apnoea
- liver disease
- kidney disease
- osteoarthritis.

What is being done about it?

The government is rolling out a number of initiatives to reduce obesity, especially in children.

- The introduction of a soft drinks industry levy.
- Investment into school programmes to encourage physical activity and healthy eating.
- Reducing the sugar content of products by 20%.
- Supporting businesses to make their products healthier.
- Updating the nutrient profile model.
- Making healthy food options more readily available.
- The production of programmes to ensure that children enjoy one hour of physical activity a day.
- Improving the nutritional value of food in schools.
- Producing a healthy rating for school foods.
- Labelling food more clearly.

In addition, the NHS provides relatively easy to follow guidelines about how you can improve your lifestyle to lose weight, such as the promotion of its 'Couch to 5k' running programme. The basic advice is to eat a healthier diet and carry out 2.5 to 5 hours of exercise per week.

Things to consider

- Some causes of obesity may be medical, such as hypothyroidism, so it is important to discuss obesity with a degree of empathy.
- Doctors and other healthcare professionals play an important role in developing the knowledge of people relating to the causes of obesity; avoid stating that the NHS should focus on treating disease in an interview, as this is simply not the case.

Smoking

For a long time, smoking has been known to have a negative impact on overall health. In the UK, around 6.4 million adults smoke cigarettes, and it is the leading cause of preventable illness. Summarised below are some key statistics from 2022 (the latest available at the time of writing).

- 12.9% of adults smoke: 14.6% of men and 11.2% of women.
- Smoking is more common in younger people, and is highest in the 25–34 age range.
- 27.2% of current smokers have no qualifications, while 6.5% of smokers have a degree or equivalent.
- Around 4.5 million adults currently use an e-cigarette.

That said, the number of adults who smoke cigarettes has steadily fallen from 16% in 2019 to 12.9% in 2022. Though not a statistically significant decrease, it is a 7.3% decrease in smokers compared to 2011, when 20.2% of the population smoked. This reduction is largely due to a number of measures taken to combat smoking in the past couple of decades, the most important being the ban on smoking inside public buildings, as a lot of people were suffering from second-hand smoke. In more recent years, the marketing on cigarette packaging has changed to include no branding, just a health warning.

There has also been a rise in 'vaping' as an alternative to smoking. In recent years, the coronavirus pandemic has also contributed to a decrease in smoking prevalence, as well as the increased usage of e-cigarettes. However, there is now increasing awareness that vaping is not the safe alternative to smoking that it was initially deemed to be. In October 2023, the government launched a consultation on youth vaping that sets out plans to reduce its appeal, affordability and availability. Similarly, the Prime Minister set out plans to create a 'smoke-free generation', by prohibiting the legal sale of cigarettes to anyone turning 14 this year or younger.

There have been some significant efforts by the NHS and Public Health England to deter individuals from smoking. You might want to look into:

- the NHS's Stop Smoking Services
- Office for Health Improvement and Disparities' Stoptober campaign.

Things to consider

- The potential health implications of vaping.
- Smoking is linked to conditions such as lung cancer, dementia and coronary artery disease, but some controversial research suggests that it could reduce the risk of Parkinson's disease and obesity. Consider the implications of this information being publicly available.

Opinions should be balanced and acknowledge the preferences of everyone; don't think purely from a medical practitioner's point of view.

Mpox

Mpox (formerly named monkeypox) is a rare infection that is most commonly found in west or central regions of Africa. In 2022 – just as the impact of Covid-19 seemed to be diminishing – cases of mpox in the UK sparked the fear of a different epidemic. Mpox is highly contagious, and is passed from person to person predominantly by physical contact with the blisters or scabs of infected individuals, touching clothing, bedding or towels that an infected person has used, or through the air droplets generated from the coughs or sneezes of an infected person who is close by. Patients infected by mpox present with symptoms such as fever, headache, muscle aches, backache, swollen lymph glands, chills, exhaustion and joint pain initially, before developing a characteristic rash, usually around the mouth, genitals and anus. Until the scabs have fallen off, leaving intact skin underneath, an infected person is contagious.

In October 2022, there were 3,673 confirmed mpox cases in the UK. Although there was a worrying surge in cases initially, the number of cases gradually declined. The main reason for the slowing of the spread was the rollout of a vaccination programme, targeting those who were most at risk for infection and transmission. In May 2023, WHO declared the global mpox emergency over.

A source of contention has been the management of mpox by the UK government. Given its transmission was predominantly between men who are gay, bisexual or have sex with other men, the Terrence Higgins Trust, a HIV and sexual health charity, was critical of the UK Health Security Agency's response, which they did not feel sufficiently targeted these high risk groups or educated them on the risks.

Artificial intelligence

Artificial intelligence is a field that incites both admiration and fear in the general population. While the risk of robots taking over is a notion that many deem to be a not too distant reality, it is impossible to ignore the great advances that developments in artificial intelligence have allowed for. Artificial intelligence refers to the use of algorithms and computer software to carry out processes that typically require human cognition, such as the ability to make inferences, deductions and decisions, as well as identifying patterns and deviations. The latter is the basis of diagnosis in many cases, which demonstrates the space for artificial intelligence in medicine.

If humans trained as doctors are able to carry out these processes, why would we want to implement machines that can do it for us? There are a number of reasons, including the following.

- **Improvements in diagnosis.** Computers are able to identify more subtle variations than humans. If disease can be spotted by identifying minor changes on an x-ray before they become apparent to the human eye, for example, it can lead to an earlier diagnosis. Subsequently, interventions will be more rapid and improved.
- **Virtual investigations.** Patients can wear devices that monitor certain outputs, and these can be monitored by 'virtual nurses', or robots, which interpret the information and contact the patient in their own home. A useful example is reminding elderly patients to take their medications at specific times, which minimises lapses in health and ultimately, hospital admissions.

- **Robotic surgery.** In recent years, there has been a considerable increase in the number of routine operations that are conducted by robotic arms. On the whole, the operations are conducted effectively and are typically associated with more rapid recovery times and fewer complications.

While artificial intelligence clearly has a place in medicine, you might want to consider possible issues. At present, the general public does not seem receptive to the idea that robots should replace healthcare professionals in any context, but would reduced waiting times for seeing a GP or having an operation change their minds? Similarly, it could save the NHS a lot of money, which could then be reallocated to areas that need it more. However, this might be accompanied by a loss of jobs in the future, which is another concern.

Current use of artificial intelligence in medicine

Some of the uses of artificial intelligence that you might want to consider further include:

- the use of nanorobots for drug delivery
- the development of electronic health records
- the analysis of test results, such as medical image scans
- digital consultations
- virtual nursing
- precision medicine
- health monitoring.

Antibiotic resistance

As bacteria are finding more ways of adapting and surviving antibiotics, the effectiveness of antibiotics is decreasing at a rapid rate. In 2018, Public Health England launched a campaign called Keep Antibiotics Working, to urge patients to only use antibiotics when absolutely required; if they are used at less critical moments, the antibiotics may not be able to counteract a more virulent illness in the future. However, it is not just the responsibility of the patient to take antibiotics as prescribed (and not save them for another illness); it is also the responsibility of doctors to appropriately prescribe them, and this is currently being addressed with doctors.

Factors that have contributed to the antibiotics resistance crisis include:

- overuse of antibiotics for cases where they are not required
- antibiotics being prescribed incorrectly
- widespread use of antibiotics in agriculture
- barriers in the pharmaceutical industry.

As well as measures being put in place to prevent the worsening of the situation, a vast amount of research is being conducted into alternative drug therapies, such as the use of monoclonal antibodies, rather than the use of antibiotics. Many of the new aims of pharmaceutical development are aligned with the concept of personalised medicine. At this time, antibiotic resistance is one of the greatest threats to the safety of patients in Europe and needs careful stewardship to ensure the effectiveness of the drugs in the next decade.

Things to consider

In recent years, there have been several outbreaks of 'incurable' infections due to the worsening of the antibiotic resistance situation. Notable cases include:

- Methicillin-resistant Staphylococcus aureus (MRSA), which ravaged hospitals over a decade ago, but is now effectively managed
- 'Super' gonorrhoea, which is a notable outbreak of an 'incurable' form of the sexually transmitted infection that became resistant to the commonly used antibiotic.

Sepsis

Sepsis is a life-threatening extreme reaction to a bodily infection; the immune system goes into overdrive and begins to damage the body's own tissues and organs. This can lead to multiple organ failure and, if not identified and treated rapidly, can lead to death. It can arise from any infection and is indiscriminate in who is affected. Its severity lies in the fact that its symptoms are often masked by or attributed to the existing infection, and there is no single diagnostic test. It can also present differently in adults and children. As such, it could be readily missed by doctors. The UK Sepsis Trust reports that five people die with sepsis every hour in the UK.

It affects 2,000 children in the UK each year. In September 2023, the health secretary announced his backing of Martha's Rule, a new piece of legislation stating that patient's have the right to a second opinion. The rule is named after Martha Mills, aged 13, who had been admitted to hospital after falling off her bike and sustaining a 'serious but survivable' injury to her pancreas. Sadly, Martha contracted an infection in hospital and died within days from sepsis. Her mother's concerns were dismissed at the time and Martha's symptoms were attributed to the side effects of her injuries. After an inquest found that a more prompt referral could have saved Martha's life, her parents called for patients to be given the right to an urgent second opinion.

Spotting sepsis

Spotting sepsis is tricky in both adults and children. In adults, symptoms may include slurred speech, extreme shivering, muscle pain, not passing urine, severe breathlessness and mottled or discoloured skin. In children, symptoms may include rapid breathing, fits or convulsions, looking mottled, bluish or pale, having a rash that does not fade when pressed, lethargy or being difficult to wake or feeling abnormally cold to the touch. In children under the age of five, symptoms may include not feeding, not passing urine or repeated vomiting.

Top 10 causes of death in the world

Around the world, the most common causes of death vary considerably depending on the country in question. A number of factors influence the situation, such as the economic stability, geographical location and healthcare provisions. The following conditions are attributed to being the most significant causes of death globally in 2019 according to the WHO, and accounted for 55% of the 55.4 million deaths that occurred in that year.

- Ischaemic heart disease, caused by the narrowing of the coronary arteries that supply the heart muscle with blood, which was responsible for around 9.5 million deaths.
- Stroke, which arises due to a blocking of the arteries that supply the brain with blood, which was responsible for just under 6 million deaths.
- Chronic obstructive pulmonary disease (COPD), such as emphysema, asthma and bronchitis, claimed 3 million lives.
- Lower respiratory infections, such as pneumonia, were the most deadly communicable disease, causing 3 million deaths.
- Neonatal conditions were responsible for the deaths of 2 million newborns in 2019, but this number has been decreasing significantly.
- Alzheimer's disease and other dementias were responsible for over 2 million deaths.
- Trachea, bronchus and lung cancers accounted for 1.8 million deaths.
- Diarrhoeal diseases contributed to 1.5 million deaths, which was a considerable decrease of 1 million since the year 2000.
- Diabetes mellitus, a chronic disease characterised by the inability to regulate blood glucose concentration, was responsible for 1.6 million deaths, which was a considerable increase since 2000.
- Kidney diseases have risen to 10th position from 13th, causing 1.3 million deaths in 2019.

Notable changes to the list of the top 10 causes of death is the removal of HIV and AIDS, as well as their related complications. This can be attributed to the improved knowledge surrounding the transmission of HIV, and individuals taking the necessary precautions, such as practising safe sex, to minimise the risk of transmission. Similarly, the availability of drugs to treat HIV has prolonged the lives of those with an infection, and it is extremely rare that these individuals develop AIDS. Most treatments reduce virus levels in the blood to undetectable levels, making it untransmissible.

Things to consider

In the UK, pre-exposure prophylaxis (PrEP), a tablet containing the drugs used to treat HIV, is readily available. By taking one tablet a day with minimal side effects, HIV negative individuals at risk of coming into sexual contact with a person with HIV can resist infection, making it an excellent way of reducing transmission. However, there are some issues associated with PrEP. The biggest issue is its association with kidney disease, so those taking it must undergo regular kidney function tests, and those with existing kidney conditions may not be able to take it. Similarly, if someone is unaware that they are HIV positive and takes a break from PrEP, they may develop drug-resistant HIV.

TIP!

It is worth looking at the ways that these diseases can be controlled, treated and prevented, highlighting any key actions that have been put in place, or any specific reasons that they cause death so frequently.

Legal cases

While medicine is a career that is incredibly rewarding, there is no doubt that it can be very stressful, and many of these situations can be attributed to the significant responsibility that a doctor carries in the care of their patients, the enormous pressures placed upon them when considering the current state of the NHS, and the questions and cases to which there are no clear answers. There have been a number of high-profile cases in recent years, and some of these are discussed below.

The Bawa-Garba case

In a ruling in 2015, Dr Bawa-Garba was convicted of manslaughter on the grounds of gross negligence following the death of a patient for whom he was responsible.

- A six-year-old patient, with Down's syndrome and a known heart condition, Jack Adcock, was admitted to Leicester Royal Infirmary on 18 February 2011 with diarrhoea, vomiting and breathing difficulties.
- He was treated by Dr Hadiza Bawa-Garba, a specialist registrar in her sixth year of training, who had an impeccable record.
- She ordered blood tests and a chest x-ray. Upon reviewing the results of the x-ray, once she was informed that they were available after a delay of several hours, Dr Bawa-Garba prescribed antibiotics for the treatment of pneumonia that were later given by nurses. The results of the blood test, which identified the presence of C-reactive protein, an indicator of infection, were not available until much later due to a technological failing.
- When debriefing with her superior, she raised her findings but did not express major concern or ask the consultant to intervene since Jack appeared to be much improved.
- When writing up her notes, Dr Bawa-Garba failed to include that Jack's medication for his heart condition should be stopped. Jack was subsequently given his medication.
- An hour later, a crash call went out and, among other doctors, Dr Bawa-Garba responded as Jack suffered cardiac arrest. As she had confused Jack with another patient, she mistakenly called off resuscitation.The mistake was recognised shortly afterwards and resuscitation continued within a few minutes.
- Shortly afterwards, Jack passed away, though it was clear that the resuscitation error was not responsible.

Other areas worthy of consideration include the fact that Dr Bawa-Garba had recently returned from maternity leave, and this was her first shift in an acute ward since returning. Prior to that fateful day, Dr Bawa-Garba's record was outstanding. However, Dr Bawa-Garba's mistakes were not the only ones worth considering, as she was failed by the hospital itself.

Below are some of the arguments in Dr Bawa-Garba's defence.

- The understaffing of the hospital meaning that Dr Bawa-Garba was extremely overworked and conducting the work of two doctors.
- There were times during the day when, despite being a trainee herself, Dr Bawa-Garba was the most senior member of staff on the ward, so she had no one to report to.
- There was no system in the hospital for the communication of results to Dr Bawa-Garba, which delayed the treatment.
- The failing of the computer systems, which prevented Dr Bawa-Garba from getting the results of the blood test in good time.
- Dr Bawa-Garba did not administer Jack's heart condition medication.

After being convicted of manslaughter, Dr Bawa-Garba had an appeal denied in 2016. There was an outcry from many doctors who felt that she was not defended appropriately, and more of an onus should have been placed on the poor working conditions in the NHS and especially, the lack of support available for junior and trainee doctors.

The failed appeal meant that Dr Bawa-Garba was struck off from the GMC register for 12 months, and this initiated a controversial series of legal events. The GMC applied to have her permanently struck off the register, but the Medical Practitioners Tribunal Services (MPTS) claimed that the punishment would be disproportionate. Unsatisfied with this response, the GMC took the MPTS to court and won, resulting in the prevention of Dr Bawa-Garba from practising medicine again. Again, this led to an enormous protest by doctors and ultimately, a crowdfunding effort that provided her with the funds to appeal her case. After a trying few years, Dr Bawa-Garba won her case, and the 12-month suspension was reinstated.

While complex, the case calls into question some of the darker aspects of working as a doctor in the NHS. As a doctor, you are responsible for your actions, even when training. For many, it is an unsettling and unpleasant side of a career in healthcare, but it is worth your reflection.

Things to consider

- What are your thoughts on this? Consider the arguments from all angles.
- If the hospital was better staffed, would Jack have died?
- If the hospital computer systems had not failed, would interventions have been faster?
- Should Dr Bawa-Garba have to take full responsibility for this case?
- Were Dr Bawa-Garba's mistakes inexcusable?

In many other jobs, a series of mistakes such as these might go unnoticed, but as a doctor, the impacts will almost always be significant.

Simon Bramhall: The liver branding surgeon

Simon Bramhall was a leading surgeon in the field of liver transplantation. He was a highly regarded surgeon owing to his fastidious approach to surgery, and as a result, he had been able to save countless lives.

Following one of these life-saving operations – a perfectly executed liver transplant – a follow-up operation was required for unrelated reasons. A different surgeon conducted the operation, and on doing so, found the 'branding' of Dr Bramhall's initials on the liver of the patient. The branding process, which used an argon beam machine typically used to control bleeding during surgery, did not damage the liver in any way.

The case was taken to trial, and was the first of its kind. Dr Bramhall admitted to two counts of assault by beating and consequently resigned from his high-profile job. During the trial, it was considered that

Dr Bramhall was tired and stressed, and during a period of significant cognitive overload, his judgement might have been impaired. However, the act was viewed as 'arrogant', and while intended to relieve tension in an overwrought operating theatre, there were considerable ethical implications.

The end result was that Dr Bramhall was fined £10,000 and made to carry out 120 hours of unpaid community service. The case divided the public, and especially his patients; some felt abused by his misuse of power, while others stated that they would be proud to have been branded by him after he saved their lives. Irrespective of personal viewpoints, it was an important case for the NHS as it reinstated patient confidence.

Case study

Dr Simon Bramhall qualified as a doctor in 1988, and held numerous prestigious positions before becoming a high profile liver transplant specialist. The complex case discussed above impeded his career, but his reflections here are worthy of your consideration.

'Once I had qualified in 1988, I worked as a house officer at a hospital in Birmingham. I also worked as an anatomy demonstrator and during that time, I trained as a surgeon. I then worked in the accident and emergency department before undertaking a surgical house officer role. I gradually worked my way up the ladder of responsibility, working as a fellowship registrar, obtaining Fellowship of the Royal College of Surgeons (FRCS). As I wasn't sure what I wanted to do at the time, I undertook a research job in the molecular study of pancreatic cancer.

'I later became a full-time lecturer in surgery and during that time, I also completed my Certificate of Completion Specialist Training (CCST). By this stage, I knew I wanted to be a liver transplant surgeon, but there were no jobs available. My post as a lecturer continued until a consultant post became available, which I was successful in obtaining. I became a high profile local, national and international liver transplant surgeon until I made a significant error during a period of enormous cognitive overload. My mistakes played out in the national and international press for a period of five years.

'During this time, I resigned from my prestigious job. I was able to continue the practice of medicine, and moved to a small Trust where I now work as a general surgeon, and support with the development of medical students as it is also a teaching hospital.

'My main areas of interest remain predominantly in liver transplant and hepato-pancreato-biliary surgery, though these are now academic interests only, as well as upper gastrointestinal tract and general surgery.

'The most rewarding aspect of my job are the patients. However, the politics that surround medicine at this time are unpleasant. The lack of resources, capacity and at times, the overregulation of our working lives, makes working in the NHS challenging.

'My biggest tip for aspiring doctors is to always be careful of your actions and to protect yourself, as what you may regard as trivial can be taken out of context. You should also ensure that you have a thorough support network, and to make sure that you give yourself a life outside of your career in medicine, as it is easy to be consumed by it.'

Things to consider

The case of Dr Bramhall raised some important concerns and areas of consideration. You might want to think about the following points.

- The patient was entirely unharmed, and it would never have been revealed if it wasn't for unrelated complications.
- Dr Bramhall and several nurses with whom he worked claimed it was merely to relieve tension, reflecting on the working conditions.
- Some people feel that the claims of abuse are extreme, but damage was inflicted on the patient without their consent.
- The patients were in a position of vulnerability as they were under general anaesthetic.
- Irrespective of how trivial an act is, there are significant consequences when it calls into question an abuse of power.

The Charlie Gard case: Great Ormond Street Hospital v Yates and Gard

The Charlie Gard case was an incredibly high-profile case in the UK during 2017. It involved Charlie Gard, an infant patient with a rare genetic disorder known as mitochondrial DNA depletion syndrome, which leads to progressive muscle and brain degeneration. Typically, the disease is fatal in infancy because of no available treatment.

The case became controversial as the parents wished to pursue alternative treatment methods, and the medical staff at Great Ormond Street Hospital (GOSH) did not believe that this was in Charlie's best interest.

The case proceeded as follows.

- Charlie was admitted to hospital in October 2016 due to shallow breathing and failure to thrive.
- Charlie was diagnosed with mitochondrial DNA depletion syndrome.
- Dr Hirano, a neurologist from New York, was working on an experimental treatment at the time and was contacted. He agreed that they should try the treatment.

- In January 2017, Charlie underwent a series of seizures that caused significant brain damage. GOSH medical staff determined that further treatment would not be beneficial and recommended palliative care.
- The parents disagreed with this view and raised the funds to transport Charlie to New York for further treatment.
- The High Court supported GOSH and overturned the parents' right to take Charlie to New York for further treatment.
- The parents appealed the case to the Court of Appeal, the Supreme Court and the European Court of Human Rights.
- The courts declined these appeals, ruling that it would be in Charlie's best interests to die with dignity.
- Several medical professionals from around the world signed a letter suggesting that controversial and unpublished data showed that the therapy could improve Charlie's condition.
- GOSH called for a new hearing in light of the evidence. Dr Hirano flew over from America to assess Charlie's condition and claimed it was too late for the therapy to be effective as Charlie's condition had deteriorated too rapidly.
- Charlie's parents abandoned legal proceedings so that they could cherish the time that they had left with him. Charlie was transferred to a hospice and life support was withdrawn.

This was a case that caught the attention of the general public, not only in the UK but around the world. The case was incredibly divisive. Some individuals felt that Charlie should be allowed to die with dignity, rather than being caused further pain through experimental medication. Others felt that his parents had a right to fight for their child's life.

Things to consider

While incredibly sensitive, there were many lessons to be learned from the Charlie Gard case. Things to consider include the following.

- The rights that parents have when considering which actions to take for their child – should the wishes of the parents be overruled by medical professionals?
- Access to experimental medicine – should parents be able to access it if they wish, even in the absence of significant evidence? If a patient is going to die anyway, should it be withheld?
- Even with the treatment, Charlie's condition would not improve, but its progression would slow down. Is it ethical to prolong the life of an individual without cognition and experiencing pain? Is it ethical to not do so?
- Should decisions be made by the courts? Should there be a fairer, faster way of resolving medical disputes?

The Charlie Gard case highlights the complex nature of medical ethics. Ethics is not personal opinion, it is a system of moral principles that demands rational reasoning and careful reflection on individual issues.

The Archie Battersbee Case: Dance and Battersbee v Barts Health NHS Trust and another

In 2022, another high-profile case was covered by the media. This time, the patient was 12-year-old Archie Battersbee, who was found unconscious by his mother after an accident that had led to cardiac arrest, causing brain damage.

The controversial element of this case came from conflicts between the wishes of Archie's parents and the medical team treating him at Royal London Hospital. Archie's parents refused to give permission for brainstem testing, to establish whether he was brainstem dead, which tends to result in a grave prognosis for the affected patient. Barts Health NHS Trust commenced legal proceedings by applying to the High Court of Justice to seek a ruling as to the lawfulness of testing, and to establish whether it was in Archie's best interests to continue receiving assistance with ventilation. Their position was that Archie had no chance of recovery due to brainstem death, and that his treatment should therefore be stopped. Archie's parents opposed these legal requests, stating that he needed more time to heal and that it would go against Archie's own religious beliefs, and sought legal support from the Christian Legal Centre and the Children and Family Court Advisory and Support Service.

The first application from Barts Health NHS Trust regarding brainstem testing was made under the Children Act 1989, which states that all decisions made on behalf of children must put their welfare first; this Act was ultimately used by the courts in ruling that Archie's treatment should end.

All medical legal cases are incredibly fraught and, as may be expected, public opinion was very divided over Archie's fate. The complexity of such cases and decisions cannot be underestimated. Disputes between families and clinical teams must ultimately be decided by the courts, and the contrast between the careful deliberation of a healthcare team and legal arbitration is very stark. All medical decisions must be made with a view to sustaining life, so a final ruling of removing life support is decided on the basis that prolonging life would be somehow harmful or would not allow for the enabling of life. Archie's case was no different, and while some firmly believed that prolonging his life would only permit greater suffering, others felt that his parents should have been allowed to decide on his behalf. These ethical debates will always exist in medicine.

The Lucy Letby case: R v Letby

The idea that a qualified nurse could intentionally cause harm to their patients, especially those who are especially vulnerable, is one that is incomprehensible to most. In 2023, the media reported on one of the most harrowing medical cases in history. Lucy Letby, formerly a neonatal nurse at the Countess of Chester Hospital, was sentenced to a whole life order for the murder of seven babies and the attempted murder of a further six babies. This makes Letby the most prolific serial killer of children in recent British history.

Letby started working at the Countess of Chester Hospital in 2012, following the completion of her nursing studies. In 2015, she undertook further training that allowed her to work with the most vulnerable and unwell babies on the high-dependency and intensive care units. Several months after Letby started in this new role, in June 2015, three babies who were otherwise healthy, despite being premature, died in quick succession, while a fourth baby's condition rapidly deteriorated and they required resuscitation – all under the supervision of Letby. In the aftermath of these events, which occurred within a two-week window, the head of the neonatal ward instructed the undertaking of an internal review, but no suspicions were raised at this point.

Between August and October 2015, another baby died suddenly, and three more babies collapsed and recovered, two of which did so several times. It was in October 2015 that senior doctors working on the ward noticed the pattern between the deterioration of babies and Letby's presence. Though they raised these concerns with senior management, they were dismissed. In February 2016, after sudden and unexpected deaths of five babies, and six others coming close to death, an external review was conducted. This review failed to identify a source of the increased mortality rates, but pointed out significant gaps in nursing and medical rotas with insufficient senior cover.

With the focus shifted away from Letby, a series of events followed between April and June 2016, with the death of one baby and deterioration and recovery of three more. In July 2016, hospital nurses associated with these cases were told that, as part of an external review, they would receive 'individual clinical supervision'. As part of this process, Letby agreed to be the first to get the supervision, and she was removed from the neonatal unit. Nevertheless, Letby put in a formal complaint about her treatment in September 2016. The chief executive of the hospital ordered the doctors who had raised concerns against Letby to apologise to her, and she was allowed to return to work.

In May 2017, the Countess of Chester Hospital NHS Foundation Trust issued a statement, saying that they had reviewed the case as thoroughly as possible, and that they were now handing over to Cheshire Police to 'seek assurances that enable [the hospital] to rule out unnatural causes of death'. The outcome of the police investigation led to Letby's arrest in July 2018 on suspicion of eight murders and six attempted murders, though she was released on bail. In June 2019, she was arrested for a second time, on suspicion of eight murders and nine attempted murders, and was once again bailed. In November 2020, Letby was arrested for the third and final time, and charged with eight counts of murder and ten counts of attempted murder. Having been denied bail on this occasion, she remained in police custody until her trial, which commenced in October 2022. Letby pleaded not guilty to seven counts of murder and fifteen counts of attempted murder, before being found guilty on 14 of the 22 charges against her in August 2023.

Following her conviction, an inquiry into the length of time it took to identify who was responsible for the deaths was called for. While Letby was a nurse rather than a doctor, the multidisciplinary nature of hospitals and medicine in general means that doctors and nurses work together very closely and determine the culture of the hospital as a workplace. The inquiry will investigate whether anyone working alongside Letby in any capacity would have been aware of her actions, and whether they should and could have raised suspicions, and whether any suspicions that were raised were taken seriously by hospital management. It will call into question the relationships between staff at different levels, including clinicians, nurses, midwives, managers and medical professionals, and whether they contributed to this failure in any way.

The lead consultant on the neonatal ward that Letby worked on, Dr Stephen Brearey, had raised concerns in October 2015 but was ignored and made to apologise. He was then put into mediation with Letby twice, which he felt was a way for the Trust to delay the investigations that he called for, rather than taking responsibility for the events that were unfolding. He has since called for the regulation of NHS executives in the same way that medical practitioners are regulated, in order to prevent the dismissal of concerns or mistreatment of whistleblowers. Though there are whistleblowing policies within the NHS that claim to protect those who raise concerns, many workers often feel that they cannot speak up, even in cases where patient safety is compromised, due to fear of repercussions.

Whistleblowers are often the reason that medical murderers, such as Letby, are brought to light. However, given the already enormous pressures of the job, potential consequences, and the element of death associated with the job, it can be especially hard for medical staff to come forward and speak out, despite their moral duty to do so. There is hope that the awful tragedies that occurred at the hands of Letby may lead to reform of both policy and culture, with NHS managers being held to account.

Moral and ethical issues

The weighted and complex questions that have a moral and/or ethical dimension constitute a very relevant and current area that has caused large amounts of discussion – and, indeed, can often polarise opinion. Many medical students with whom we have spoken tell us that, almost without exception, either one or several of the following issues were discussed at the interview stage.

When answering questions on ethics, there are no specific answers, and each individual's answer is likely to vary slightly. It is worth applying the four pillars of ethics to your answers to ensure that they are aligned with the core principles of healthcare.

- **Autonomy.** Your actions must respect the rights of the patient, as well as their right to make decisions about their healthcare.
- **Beneficence.** Your actions must be advantageous to the patient.
- **Non-maleficence.** Your actions must not harm the patient.
- **Justice.** You must treat all patients equally.

Euthanasia and assisted deaths

Euthanasia is illegal in the UK, and doctors alleged to have given a patient a lethal dose of a medication with the intention of ending life will be charged with manslaughter or murder, depending on the circumstances surrounding each case. UK law also prohibits assisting with suicide.

However, in order to prove the offence of aiding and abetting it is necessary to prove firstly that the person in question has taken their own life and, secondly, that an individual or individuals aided and abetted the person in committing suicide.

In October 2014 the Director of Public Prosecutions (DPP) published an updated policy on prosecuting assisted suicide cases. The Crown Prosecution Service (CPS) website gives details of the public interest factors against prosecution. These include:

1. the victim had reached a voluntary, clear, settled and informed decision to commit suicide
2. the suspect was wholly motivated by compassion
3. the actions of the suspect, although sufficient to come within the definition of the offence, were of only minor encouragement or assistance
4. the suspect had sought to dissuade the victim from taking the course of action which resulted in his or her suicide
5. the actions of the suspect may be characterised as reluctant encouragement or assistance in the face of a determined wish on the part of the victim to commit suicide
6. the suspect reported the victim's suicide to the police and fully assisted them in their enquiries into the circumstances of the suicide or the attempt and his or her part in providing encouragement or assistance.

Source: www.cps.gov.uk/legal-guidance/policy-prosecutors-respect-cases-encouraging-or-assisting-suicide. Contains public sector information licensed under the Open Government Licence v3.0.

The Tony Nicklinson case in March 2012 brought this law into question. A stroke left Tony Nicklinson paralysed from the neck down and with 'locked-in syndrome'. While High Court judges sympathised with his case, they refused his appeal to grant immunity to a doctor to help him end his life, stating that it was for Parliament to decide, not the judicial process. Tony Nicklinson died of pneumonia six days after this hearing, having starved himself in response to the judgement; however, the family continue to fight this ruling for other sufferers in similar predicaments. In 2013, the Court of Appeal rejected cases from Jane Nicklinson and Paul Lamb (who was paralysed after a road accident) despite intervention from the British Humanist Association (BHA), which was seeking to lend its support. A second case was won, however, in a case for a man known only as 'Martin'. A ruling from two Court of Appeal judges said the law should be 'spelt out unambiguously' over whether those seeking to help would be prosecuted, with the DPP now forced to clarify and possibly having to state that prosecutions will not be made against those who help.

In June 2015, a Bill proposed by Lord Falconer completed its first reading in the House of Lords, but ran out of time before the 2015 General Election. If approved by both Houses of Parliament, this new law would have allowed terminally ill, mentally competent adults to request that a doctor provide them with life-ending medication, and the doctor would not face criminal prosecution for taking a positive step to help end a patient's life. The current law only allows doctors to withdraw medication and sustenance from a patient in a persistent vegetative state.

In 2015, Simon Binner again brought this issue to the media as he posted details of his condition – motor neurone disease – along with the dates of his death and funeral on his LinkedIn page, before flying to Switzerland for assisted suicide, thus continuing to raise the debate about dignity over legality. Also in 2015 the Assisted Dying Bill – the first real move to change UK law on the right to die – was overwhelmingly rejected by MPs at the second reading.

In the years since, three more cases have been rejected by the courts regarding the assisted suicide of four terminally ill patients with a life expectancy limited to months, as well as a case by a man who was paralysed in a car accident. The latter case was arguably more significant in its outcome given that his life expectancy is not limited, but he lives with chronic pain. In 2020, the media also extensively covered the story of Mavis Eccleston, an 80-year-old woman who was tried for murder and manslaughter, but cleared of all charges, after assisting her terminally ill husband in dying by providing and administering an overdose of prescription medication, which the couple had been stockpiling.

In 2021, members of the British Medical Association voted on its position on assisted dying, which it had previously opposed. The vote saw 49% of members in favour, 48% opposing and 3% abstaining, which resulted in them adopting a neutral stance. The divisive nature of the vote was disappointing to assisted dying advocates and charities, but the shift in stance could alter the way that future cases are dealt with.

In May 2021, Baroness Meacher introduced the Assisted Dying Bill to permit assisted dying for mentally competent terminally ill adults. The bill outlined that two independent doctors and a High Court judge must oversee and approve the request from such individuals considered to bein the final six months of their lives, to then permit the prescription of life-ending medication. The bill received its first reading in the House of Lords in May 2021, before being debated at its second reading in October 2021. The bill passed this stage unopposed with considerable support across parties, but ran out of time to pass all of the required stages before the end of the parliamentary session in May 2022. This has led the charity Dignity in Dying to urge political parties to amend their manifestoes to provide sufficient time for the full scrutiny of future assisted dying bills through their Make Time for Assisted Dying campaign.

Significantly, in November 2021, politicians in Jersey voted in favour of the principle of legalising assisted dying. Since then, a series of public consultations on detailed proposals has taken place, with the consultation feedback report published in April 2023. Based on this feedback, the proposals are now being refined and an ethics review will be undertaken. From late 2023, the proposals will be debated by the States Assembly and, if approved, law drafting will begin in 2024. The consequences of these events in Jersey could ultimately impact the laws on assisted dying far beyond the island.

Campaigners for assisted dying are hopeful that 2024 will see real progress in legislation in favour of their cause across the British Isles.

Things to consider

When answering questions on euthanasia, consider the following.

- Discuss the fact that euthanasia is complex; there are no black and white answers, which makes drawing conclusions difficult.
- Discuss the legal aspects of euthanasia: assisted suicide or active euthanasia is illegal in the UK, but there are other countries where either of these acts, or both of them, are legal. As such, it is worth keeping an eye on any changes in the law.
- Reflect on the ethical considerations: it appeals to the beneficence ethical pillar, yet contrasts with the concept of non-maleficence.
- The ethical guidelines provided by the GMC must ultimately be relied upon.
- Any other factors, such as the mental capacity of the patient and any pressures that may have been applied, must also be rigorously investigated.

Do not fall into the trap of giving your personal opinion, and falling on one side of the argument. It is crucial that you make use of the four pillars of ethics.

Abortion

Even recently there was new controversy regarding abortion, as the BMA issued guidance advising doctors that 'there may be circumstances in which termination of pregnancy on foetal grounds would be lawful'. As reported in the *Telegraph*, there was a backlash from MPs who criticised the BMA for trying to redefine abortion laws. In the wake of the controversial decision of the CPS not to prosecute two doctors who were secretly filmed offering to abort selected-sex babies, the DPP warned that the guidance for doctors needs urgently to be updated. The current BMA guidance suggests that it is 'unethical' to terminate a pregnancy on the grounds of sex alone, but it also says that the wishes and situation of the mother should be considered. The Law and Ethics of Abortion BMA Views report of November 2014 says that in England, Scotland and Wales, provided the criteria from the Abortion Act 1967 are fulfilled, then abortion is lawful. It goes on to say that unless it is necessary to save the life of the mother, doctors have a right to conscientious objection should they wish.

One in three women will have an abortion before they are 45 years old, and in 2021 there were 214,256 abortions in England and Wales. Yet, without certain conditions being met, abortion is still illegal. Indeed, it has long been the subject of controversy in Northern Ireland, where it was only decriminalised in October 2019.

Abortion is a highly divisive topic, and in recent years, anti-abortion activists have become increasingly prevalent, leading to a parliamentary decision to introduce buffer zones in the immediate vicinity surrounding abortion facilities, banning any behaviour that could be considered to be protesting in an attempt to prevent the influencing or intimidation of patients. These buffer zones came into effect in Northern Ireland in September 2023, following the introduction of the Abortion Services (Safe Access Zones) Act (Northern Ireland) 2023. Anti-abortion protests outside some specific abortion clinics is now a criminal offence that is punishable by a fine.

Things to consider

As with any ethical topic, abortion is a complex area with no clear cut answers. When discussing it, you should consider the following points.

- Outline that it is a controversial issue.
- Discuss the legal aspects – that abortion is legal in the UK up to 24 weeks of pregnancy following the agreement of two doctors that the abortion would be less damaging to the woman's physical and mental health than the pregnancy itself. In rare medical instances, it is legal for abortions to take place after this date.
- When considering the four pillars of ethics, autonomy states that patients have a right to make decisions about their bodies.

- Beneficence suggests that doctors must prioritise the best interests of the patient, which in this case would be the mother, whose mental and physical well-being must be considered.
- Non-maleficence raises possibly the most controversial aspect. While abortion may cause harm to the patient, it also raises questions about the sanctity of human life. On the whole, it is a complex and sensitive element, so regardless of personal opinion, it is best not to dwell on this for too long.
- Again, refer to the ethical guidelines provided by the GMC.

Refusal of treatment

As per the ethical pillar of patient autonomy, patients have the right to make decisions about their own treatment. Before a medical intervention is conducted, patients must give consent, and this is the case for all procedures, ranging from a straightforward blood test to a complex operation.

For a patient to rightfully refuse treatment, the decision must be entirely voluntary, and not a result of coercion by another party, such as a relative or a healthcare professional. In addition, the patient must make the decision in a manner that is informed; they must have a thorough understanding of what the treatment is for, what it entails, possible alternatives and consequences of going through with the refusal.

While patient decisions must be respected, there is an exception to this rule and refusal of treatment can be overturned if the doctor in charge of the patient's care feels that the patient lacks the capacity to make an informed and voluntary decision. In this instance, capacity refers to the ability to demonstrate an understanding of the decision and an ability to communicate it with the healthcare professionals. For the most part, adults are deemed to be capable of making informed and voluntary decisions, but some conditions may influence this, including:

- those with dementia
- those affected by mental health conditions, such as schizophrenia or bipolar disorder
- those under the influence of drugs or alcohol.

Another area of consideration includes advance decisions. Individuals older than 18 years of age can produce what is referred to as a 'living will', which typically details the refusal of future medical interventions, in the case that they might be incapable of making those decisions at the time. One example is the signing of Do Not Attempt Resuscitation (DNAR) forms so that life-saving interventions are not utilised in the case of cardiac arrest.

Things to consider

As with other ethical issues, when discussing refusal of treatment, you must consider all of the ethical arguments associated with the issue.

- Consider the role of the doctor in this situation – they must fully inform the patient of what the treatment is, what it entails, whether there are alternative treatments and the consequences of not accepting the treatment.
- When considering the four pillars of ethics, patient autonomy must be respected.
- The doctor also has a role in assessing the capability of a patient in making the decision, and ensuring that the decision is not being influenced by a third party.
- Beneficence in this situation would be to provide the patient with the treatment that they require.
- However, if this is against the patient's wishes, then it may be that giving the treatment will do more harm than it will good, thereby conflicting with the non-maleficence pillar of ethics.
- Finally, refer to the GMC's guidelines on the situation.

Other ethical questions

The ethical considerations in medicine are extensive, and you should research as many as possible. As a starting point, you should consider some of the following points.

- A patient is diagnosed with Huntington's disease, but does not want to pass the information on to his children, from whom he is estranged.
- The importance of patient confidentiality when dealing with a child.
- The NHS should not fund treatment for obesity-related diseases.
- You witness a colleague being rude and offensive to a patient.
- You are working as a doctor and your colleague and friend, also a practising doctor, turns up to work under the influence of alcohol.
- You have two patients who require a liver transplant and a liver becomes available that suits both of them. One is an ex-alcoholic mother with two young children while the other is a teenager who was born with a liver defect. Who do you give it to?

Remember, not all ethical scenarios will be directly related to medicine. They may ask you about something entirely unrelated to assess your reaction, so don't be surprised if this happens at interview!

TIP!

Useful documents to review when preparing for medical school interviews:

- *Tomorrow's Doctors*, provided by the General Medical Council
- *Medical Ethics Today*, provided by the British Medical Association

8 | Results day

The A level results will arrive at your school on the third Thursday in August. For International Baccalaureate (IB) qualifications results day will be in the first week of July and for students studying in Scotland it will be the first week of August. The medical schools will have received them a few days earlier. You must make sure that you are at home on the day the results are published and able to travel in to your school or college to collect them. If you are unable to do this, speak to your school or college about making arrangements for your results to be given to you by email as early as possible on the day, if they don't automatically do so; don't wait for the school to post the results slip to you. If you need to act to secure a place, you may have to do so quickly. This chapter will take you through the steps you should take after receiving your results and also explains what to do if your grades are below what you expected.

If things go wrong during the exams

If something happens when you are preparing for or actually taking the exams that prevents you from doing your best, you must notify your school/college as soon as possible. They should then notify the exam board and the medical schools that have made you offers. Ensure that these parties are made aware of your situation as soon as possible; it is no good waiting for disappointing results and then telling everyone that you were ill at the time but said nothing to anyone. Exam boards can give you special consideration if the appropriate forms are sent to them by the school, along with supporting evidence. An increasing number of medical schools now only accept mitigating circumstances if they were reported to the exam board at the time of the examination.

Your extenuating circumstances must be significant. Feeling slightly under the weather won't do! If you are ill to the extent that you are unable to prepare for the exams or to perform effectively during them, it is a good idea to consult your GP and obtain a letter describing your condition.

The other main cause of underperformance is distressing events at home. If a member of your immediate family is very seriously ill, or if you have some form of significant domestic disruption, you should explain this to your head teacher and ask him or her to write to the exam boards and medical schools. However, the vast majority of universities now expect that extenuating circumstances are taken into account by the exam boards, and the allowance would have been given in terms of the final mark adjustment by the board. You can by all means contact the medical school to discuss on results day, but they are likely to have already taken it in to account by that point. The extenuating circumstances might allow reapplication to universities that usually don't usually take retakes.

The medical school admissions departments are well organised and efficient, but they are staffed by human beings. If there were extenuating circumstances that could have affected your exam performance and that were brought to their notice in June, it is a good idea to ask them to review the relevant letters shortly before the exam results are published.

If you hold an offer and get the grades

If you previously received a conditional offer and your grades equal or exceed that offer, congratulations! You can relax and wait for your chosen medical school to send you joining instructions. One word of warning: you cannot assume that grades of A*AB satisfy an AAA offer. This is especially true if the B grade is in biology or chemistry. You should call your chosen university as soon as possible to check if you have met your offer.

If you have good grades but no offer

Very few schools keep places open and, of those that do, most will choose to allow applicants who hold a conditional offer to slip a grade rather than dust off a reserve list of those they interviewed but didn't make an offer to. They are even less likely to consider applicants who appear out of the blue, no matter how high their grades are. In recent years, a small number of universities have offered Clearing places. With the increased number of places being made available for studying medicine at university, it is possible that more spaces will be available through Clearing, although this is not an option that should be relied upon.

If you hold three A grades or above but were rejected when you applied through UCAS, you need to let the medical schools know that you are out there. The best way to do this is by phone and email. Places available to students in this position are few and far between, so it is preferable to phone in order to make contact as quickly as possible. Contact details are listed in the UCAS directory and are on the university websites.

Set out overleaf is sample text for an email, which can also be used as the basis of a phone call. Make sure you write your own version of this; don't copy it word for word!

To: Mrs Lister

Subject: Application to study medicine at Rushmere University

Dear Mrs Lister

UCAS no. 16-024680-8

I applied to study medicine at Rushmere University this year. I regrettably was rejected as a result of my interview/without an interview, which at the time I was disappointed to hear. Today I received grades:

Biology – A
Chemistry – A*
Maths – A*

While I appreciate this is a very busy time of year for you and that it is non-standard to take applicants at this stage of the year, I am contacting you to see if, after results day, there were any places still at Rushmere University to study medicine. I learned a great deal from my interview experience previously and I would be very willing to attend another interview at short notice to demonstrate that I have taken on board the advice I was given.

I look forward to hearing from you.

Yours sincerely,

Charlotte Stevenson

If, despite your most strenuous efforts, you are unsuccessful, you need to consider applying again (see below). The other alternative is to use the Clearing system to obtain a place on a degree course related to medicine and prepare to apply again once you have completed your first degree.

If you hold an offer but miss the grades

If you have only narrowly missed the required grades, you can contact the medical school to put your case forward. Most universities will have made their decision in advance of results day and are unlikely to be swayed; however, there is nothing to be lost by trying. Sample text for another email follows below.

To: Mrs Lister

Subject: Application to study medicine at Rushmere University

Dear Mrs Lister

UCAS no. 16-024680-8

I have a conditional offer to study medicine at Rushmere University this year. However, I am afraid that having received my results, I found that I have missed my offer. Today I received grades:

Biology – B
Chemistry – A
Maths – A*

As you can see, I just missed the offer by one grade in Biology, though I received a higher grade than anticipated in Maths. Therefore, I was wondering if you could guide me as to whether my grades are still applicable for my offer or what the next steps are if my offer is to be rescinded.

I look forward to hearing from you and remain resolute and determined to achieve my place at Rushmere University, as for me, it is without question where I wish to develop and train as a doctor.

Yours sincerely,

Charlotte Stevenson

If this is unsuccessful, you need to consider retaking your A levels and applying again (see below). The other alternative is to use the Clearing system to try and obtain a place on a degree course related to medicine and prepare to apply to a medical course after you graduate.

Retaking A levels

The grade requirements for retake candidates are potentially higher than for first-timers (usually A*AA). You should retake any subject where your first result was below B and you should aim for at least an A grade.

Remember that if you resit A levels under the current system, you have to take all of the exams again, with no guarantee that your grade will improve. Check with your college or school on its provisions for students wanting to retake. It is also possible to retake A levels at some further education and independent colleges. Interviews to discuss this are free and carry no obligation to enrol on a course, so it is worth taking the time to talk to their staff before you embark on A level retakes.

It is possible to resit IB examinations. This is available in either November or May, though you would have to complete them within three opportunities to complete the qualification. You can retake a Scottish Higher in a separate academic year and the same is true for Advanced Highers, but not in all subjects. You would have to register again for, and then resit, the Advanced Highers. The same applies for the IB examinations, as you would effectively need to sit the whole qualification again.

Reapplying to medical school

Many medical schools discourage retake candidates (see Table 8, pages 214–217), so the whole business of applying again needs careful thought, hard work and a bit of luck. The choice of medical schools for your UCAS application will be narrower than it was the first time round, so it is vital to carefully research which universities you will be eligible to apply to. Don't apply to the medical schools that discourage retakers unless there really are special, extenuating circumstances to explain your disappointing grades, such as:

- your own illness
- the death or serious illness of a very close relative
- serious domestic upheaval, such as divorce.

These are just guidelines; the only safe method of finding out if a medical school will accept you is to ask directly. Send an email so that you can have a record of the reply that they send. Text for a typical email is set out below. Don't follow it slavishly and do take the time to write to a wide range of medical schools before you make your final choice.

To: Mrs Lister

Subject: Application to study medicine at Rushmere University

Dear Mrs Lister

UCAS no. 16-024680-8

I am hopeful of applying to Rushmere University this year but I am retaking my A levels.

This year, I received the following grades

Biology – B
Chemistry – B
Spanish – B

I am retaking all of the above and am expected to achieve at least A grades in all subjects.

I note that you encourage retake applicants in specific circumstances; however, I am not sure if I would be eligible and I hope that you will be able to advise me. I do not have any extenuating circumstances that have affected my performance.

I look forward to hearing from you.

Yours sincerely,

Charlotte Stevenson

Make sure that your email is brief, clear and well presented, and follows the format detailed below:

- opening paragraph
- your exam results: set out clearly and with no omissions
- any extenuating circumstances: a brief statement
- your retake plan, including the timescale
- a request for help and advice
- closing formalities.

The same advice applies if you are reapplying with qualifications other than A levels. If you did not get a place but now have the grades required, then you will probably be able to reapply, but make sure you talk to the medical schools first. If you have not got the grades, then you need to look at what routes are available. If you do not resit the IB, you will need to look at A levels or Foundation programmes in order to reach the requisite entry requirements for a medicine course. If you have taken Scottish Highers, depending on the subject, you are able to retake again in a new academic year. Either way, you must make sure that you gain the necessary qualifications in the next sitting – even though this will allow entry to only a handful of medical schools, you should still make contact and speak to the admissions tutors at those medical schools that consider retakes.

Case study

Lucy has completed three years of her medicine degree, and is currently undertaking an intercalation year to gain an insight into clinical research. Lucy's studies are now well underway, but to get into medical school, she needed to retake her A levels.

'As clichéd as it sounds, I have always known I wanted to be a doctor. I always loved helping people, and all of the steps that I took along the way – work experience, working as a carer, volunteering in care homes – all confirmed it for me. Unfortunately for me, I wasn't a huge chemistry enthusiast! While there were options where you didn't have to study chemistry at A level to get into medical school, these were limited and I wanted to give myself the best chance possible. I struggled through my A levels and obtained A grades in Biology and Classics, but my B grade in Chemistry prevented me from taking up the offers that I held at Leicester and Plymouth.

'I was devastated, and for the duration of results day, I really thought it was the end of the world! I begged and pleaded on the phone to the universities, but there just wasn't any scope that year, even though some of my peers had gained their places with the same set of grades at different universities. After my initial disappointment, I started to weigh up my options. I had started to think of back-up plans well in advance of results day, and this is definitely something I would advise prospective medics to do – as horrible a prospect as it is, it can take a lot of work out of a period of time where you don't want to do anything other than cry! My back-up options were to study abroad, or undertake an alternative degree and pursue medicine as a graduate, or retake my A level exams to get the grades I needed. My research had highlighted that retaking my A levels would limit my options for applications, as not all medical schools considered retakes, but given my grades profile at first sitting, there was a decent number I could consider that would make it a worthwhile option.

'Studying chemistry again was the last thing I wanted to do, but after reviewing my options, I knew that initially this was my best plan. Now I am a bit older, the thought of studying abroad is attractive, but at the time I knew I would struggle to settle in a new country while studying something as challenging as medicine. I also knew that balancing medicine with learning a new language for placements would be too much for me. I also recognised that this option would still be there in the future if I needed it!

'I also decided against studying a different degree. I knew that many people found this advantageous in the long run, and on reflection, this could have been a very good option for me. I am now studying alongside people who did this and, especially in the first few years, they were far more prepared for university-level study than many of us. People who had studied medical or biomedical related degrees also had the upper hand with some of the taught content. Again, I knew this could be a back-up option a year down the road if my exams didn't work out.

'Part of me wanted to spend my entire year out studying chemistry, but after a couple of months of preparing only for the application and the chemistry exams, I knew I needed to do something else to keep me sane. I got a job working as a healthcare assistant and while it certainly threw me in at the deep end, it was pivotal in my development as a person, and I learned so many skills and got comfortable talking to and working with patients, families and doctors. It was an intense year as the work was physically exhausting and chemistry continued to be a hatred of mine! I reached out to my former teachers, who helped me with my application and allowed me to sit my exams (including mock exams) with them, which took a lot of stress out of the application and exam process. If anyone finds themselves in this position, I would encourage them to reach out to their former school to see how they can help. Navigating things like exam centres can be quite daunting!

'Ultimately, I got two offers to study medicine from Exeter and Southampton. I wasn't really sure how the interviews would pan out, so I was delighted to receive two offers! It really motivated me to keep pushing myself with the chemistry revision. Thankfully, it all paid off and I was able to go to my first-choice university.

'Fast forward four years and I am now intercalating at the University of Southampton. Studying medicine has been intense at times but really enjoyable. I have covered the first phase, which involves studying the body systems and some modules in the practical elements of studying medicine; and the second phase, which is based in clinical medicine. At the start of the third year, I undertook a short research project and really enjoyed it. Although it wasn't something I had planned to do or even considered, I then decided to think about intercalation. When you are surrounded by aspiring medics, you realise that everyone is on their own paths and timelines. Some people are very eager to just get through it and start practising. I had already taken a year out, and that had helped me so much that I wanted to take another opportunity to learn more widely. Research is integral to medicine, and I wanted to get my hands dirty and my brain ticking in a different way! I am only a few months into studying placental viability, but it is very different to what I am used to and I am loving it. I'm not sure what the future holds in terms of a career path, but I am definitely keeping the door open to research.

'My advice to people who want to study medicine, especially if things don't go to plan, is to keep a clear head. Despite what it might feel like, there's no rush. Medicine will always be there, so think about the best route for you. I would also encourage you to think about the opportunities that are presented to you. It is tempting to singularly focus on clinical medicine and qualifying, but it can be good to get more broad experience sometimes.'

9 | Non-standard applications

So far, this book has been concerned with the 'standard' applicant: the UK resident who is studying at least two science subjects at A level/ in the IB course/Scottish Highers – and who is applying from school or who is retaking immediately after disappointing grades. However, what about students who do not have this 'standard' background, such as international students? Or those who have not studied science A levels? The main non-standard applicants and the steps they should take to apply to medical school are outlined in this chapter.

Those who have not studied science A levels

If you decide that you would like to study medicine after having already started on a combination of A levels that does not fit the subject requirements for entry to medical school, you are potentially eligible to apply for a 'foundation' year, although at present, only the medical schools at the University of Manchester and University of Liverpool offer this route.

The course covers elements of chemistry, biology and physics and prepares you for the demands of the degree course. The pre-medical course lasts one academic year.

If your application is rejected, you will have to spend a further two years taking science A levels at a sixth-form college so that you meet the subject entry requirements of the standard course. Alternatively, some colleges offer one-year A level courses, but only very able students can cover A levels in chemistry and biology in a single year with good results. You should discuss your particular circumstances with the staff of a number of colleges in order to select the course that will prepare you to achieve the A level grades you need in the subjects you require.

Those who have faced barriers to learning

There are a number of medical schools that offer what is known as a 'Gateway Year'. This is to allow academically able students who have faced barriers to learning to gain entry onto a medical degree.

To be eligible to apply for these courses, there are specific combinations of contextual factors that have to be met. These factors are usually related to things such as living in an area of social deprivation or attending a school with low academic achievement. It is vital that you look closely at the criteria that need to be met before considering this as an option.

Overseas students

Competition for the few places available to overseas students is fierce, and you would be wise to discuss your application informally with the medical school before submitting your UCAS application. The UCAS website gives a useful overview of international student statistics that illustrate perfectly the difficulties faced by international applicants. For example, in 2022, there were a total of 108,390 applications (not applicants) for medicine, with 87,960 made by domestic students, and 20,430 made by international students. Some 9,500 domestic students and 1,215 international students were accepted.

Many medical schools give preference to students who do not have adequate provision for training in their own countries. You should contact the medical schools individually for advice on the application procedure and costs.

Following the UK's departure from the EU in January 2020 and the end of the transition period in January 2021, EU students are now treated in a similar way to non-EU international students, particularly in terms of the fees they pay. EU students are no longer eligible for home fee status or financial support from Student Finance unless they have citizens' rights or are an Irish citizen. Further details can be found at www.gov.uk/guidance/studying-in-the-uk-guidance-for-eu-students.

Graduates and mature students

Graduates

Course options available to graduates include the following:

- four-year graduate-entry courses
- five-year courses in the normal way
- some six-year pre-medical/medical courses
- Access to Medicine Diploma courses.

You should check which Access to Medicine Diploma courses are accepted by medical schools, as most will not consider them. Often, each medical school has a shortlist of Access courses from which it accepts applications, so it is important to check carefully what the individual requirements are. It is also usually the case that you have to reach a very high level of achievement in these courses, not just pass them.

Mature students

In recent years the options available for mature students have increased enormously. There is a growing awareness that older students often represent a 'safer' option for medical schools because they are likely to be more committed to medicine and less likely to drop out, and are able to bring to the medical world many skills and experiences that 18-year-olds sometimes lack. In general, there are two types of mature applicant:

1. those who have always wanted to study medicine but failed to get into medical school when they applied from school in the normal way
2. those who came to the idea later on in life, often having embarked on a totally different career.

The first type of mature applicant has usually followed a degree course in a subject related to medicine and has obtained a good grade (minimum 2.i). This pathway is well trodden and there are many medical professionals who have entered the profession via this route. The second category of mature student is those who have achieved success in other careers and who can bring a breadth of experience to the medical school and to the profession.

Options available for mature students are summarised below. The chapter then examines each option in more detail.

Applicants with A levels that satisfy medical schools' standard offers

Can apply for five-/six-year courses in the normal way.

Applicants with A levels that do not satisfy standard offers

This could include arts A levels, or grades that are too low. Applicants in this category can take the following routes.

- Retake/pick up new A levels at sixth-form college and apply for five-/six-year courses in the normal way.
- Enrol on a six-year course that includes a preliminary year. These courses are designed for students who achieved high grades at A level but did not take the required number of science subjects to apply for the A100 course. This course is available at Manchester and Liverpool, and includes a foundation (pre-medical) year designed for students with no more than one science subject at A level. This course should not be confused with the six-year (usually A100) courses offered by many medical schools that include an intercalated BSc.

- Enrol on an Access course.
- Enrol on a six-year course that includes a gateway year. These courses are designed for able students who have specific contextual factors that have impacted on their attainment and fulfil specific widening participation criteria. Before considering applying to one of these courses, you must carefully investigate their criteria to ensure that you are eligible. The courses are available at:
  - Aberdeen
  - Bristol
  - Dundee
  - Edge Hill
  - UEA
  - Glasgow
  - Hull York
  - Keele
  - King's
  - Lancaster
  - Leeds
  - Leicester
  - Lincoln
  - Liverpool
  - Nottingham
  - Plymouth
  - Southampton
  - St Andrews

Mature students with no formal A level or equivalent qualifications

Applicants in this category can take the following routes:

- A levels, then five-/six-year courses in the normal way
- Access courses (see page 180).

Preparing the application

Mature students and graduates are faced with many decisions on the route to becoming a doctor. Not only do they have to decide which course or combination of courses might be suitable, but in many cases they also have to try to gauge how best to juggle the conflicting demands of study, financial practicalities and their families.

Mature students need to prepare carefully for their applications in order to ensure that they are recognised as being fully committed to a career as a doctor. Typically, when a mature student is interviewed, the interviewers are interested in:

- why you have decided to change direction
- what you have done to convince yourself that this is the right career path
- what your career has given you in the way of personal qualities that are relevant to medicine
- what skills and personal qualities you have developed in your previous career that are relevant to medicine.

Case study

Jaideep is currently working as a Foundation Year 2 doctor after studying on a graduate entry programme. Prior to studying medicine, Jaideep studied engineering at undergraduate level and completed a PhD in biological imaging before working abroad as a surfing instructor while volunteering in care roles. Despite it being convoluted, Jaideep is appreciative of the route he took as it meant he was absolutely confident in his decision to pursue medicine.

'As a 17-year-old trying to decide what and where to study, I was completely overwhelmed, so I just opted for a subject that promised career stability and a decent salary, which is all I had ever really aspired to growing up in a working-class family.

'Engineering was an interesting first degree, and there were some elements I really enjoyed, but I didn't really see myself working as an engineer, so opted to undertake a PhD in a more medical field. I knew I didn't want to stay in academia after finishing my PhD, but wasn't entirely sure where to go next. I decided to return to my native Punjab to visit family, andended up working in basic jobs and volunteering. And it was here that I first felt that there was a job in healthcare that I might be aligned with. It was so rewarding helping in the smallest ways, and intellectually appealing. In India, the healthcare system doesn't parallel that in the UK and, as a volunteer, I wasn't guarded from the harsh realities as we might be here. Having witnessed some incredibly challenging situations in far from ideal conditions, I felt comfortable with the adversities that working in medicine might bring.

'Eventually I opted to apply to study medicine, and returned to the UK after receiving offers from several medical schools. After six years of university study, another four did feel a bit daunting, but I enjoyed every minute of it. As soon as there was patient contact, I felt right at home and knew I'd made the right decision.

'I currently work in a hospital in Hampshire as an FY2 in obstetrics and gynaecology. Babies can arrive or give their mums trouble at any time, so the shifts are long and busy, but the thrill of the work makes them go quickly. With the NHS under constant strain, there are some elements of the job that can be challenging, and, of course, any losses or difficult diagnoses can be difficult to deal with – this is one aspect of the job that I have found quite tough.

'For anyone considering medicine who perhaps isn't 100% sure, my advice would be not to rush into it. Take your time to figure out exactly what you want to do and then take it from there. Studying as a graduate was challenging financially, but there is support available if you look for it. Make sure you are thoroughly prepared for the realities of medicine rather than focusing on the ideals, but remember that the ideals make it all worth it.'

Personal statement

When writing your personal statement, try to get a number of people to read it and give you their opinion. However, the most useful opinions will come from academic staff at your school or college or doctors who have a role in recruiting students. Keep your writing simple, make sure to write in continuous prose, don't overuse the thesaurus, and check spelling and punctuation extremely carefully.

For mature applicants, the UCAS personal statement needs to be carefully structured. The strictly limited space means that a concise but convincing case has to be constructed. Full details on writing the personal statement can be found in Chapter 5.

For mature applicants, structure your personal statement as follows.

1. Why you want to study medicine.
2. Brief career and educational history.
3. Reasons for the change of direction.
4. What you have done to investigate medicine, including work experience and voluntary work.
5. Brief details of achievements, interests.

The most important thing to bear in mind is that you must convince the selectors that you are serious about the change in direction, and that your decision to apply to study medicine is not a spur-of-the-moment reaction to dissatisfaction with your current job or studies.

A useful exercise is to try to imagine that you are the person who will read the personal statement in order to decide whether to interview or to reject without interview. Does your personal statement contain sufficient indication of thorough research, preparation and long-term commitment? If it does not, you will be rejected. As a rough guide, approximately three-quarters of it should cover your reasons for applying for a medical course and the preparation and research that you have undertaken. The further back in time you can demonstrate that you started to plan your application, the stronger it will be.

The personal statement is expected to be replaced by a set of questions in future (but no earlier than the 2024/25 application cycle for 2026 entry). For more information see page 74.

Applying for a Gateway course

Gateway courses or programmes are not to be confused with Access courses. As the name suggests, these courses usually act as a 'gateway' for entering Year 1 of a standard medical course.

You will need to look at the website of each medical university to find out if it offers this course. These courses are now specifically aimed at widening participation of students from deprived backgrounds and so are not appropriate for all students. Make sure you look carefully at the eligibility details to ensure that you meet the criteria for any course you are considering applying to.

Access courses

A number of colleges of further education offer Access to Medicine courses. These courses cover biology, chemistry, physics and other medically related topics, and usually last one year. Some medical schools will accept students who have successfully completed the course, but it is important to check which universities you will be able to apply to before commencing. Contact details can be found at the end of the book.

Four-year graduate courses

Often known as Graduate Entry Programmes (GEPs), these are usually given the code A101 or A102 by UCAS. The first medical schools to introduce accelerated courses specifically for graduates were St George's Hospital Medical School and Leicester/Warwick (which has since split into two separate medical schools). Courses can be divided into two types:

1. those for graduates with a medically related degree
2. those that accept graduates with degrees in any discipline.

The following medical schools run GEPs (see www.ucas.com):

- Bangor
- Cambridge
- Cardiff
- Chester
- Dundee and St Andrews (ScotGEM)
- King's
- Newcastle
- Nottingham
- Oxford
- Queen Mary
- Sheffield
- Southampton
- St George's
- Surrey
- Swansea
- Ulster
- Warwick
- Worcester.

Graduate pre-admissions tests

The UCAT and GAMSAT (Graduate Medical School Admissions Test) are used by some graduate-entry providers for their graduate-specific medical courses. In addition, there are some universities that now use GAMSAT for graduates applying to the standard non-graduate medical course. The BMAT (BioMedical Admissions Test) was last used in 2023 for 2024 entry, and will not be used by universities going forward. At the time of writing, some universities that previously used BMAT are still deciding on their arrangements for testing in 2024. The universities using each test are summarised in Table 7 below.

Table 7 Graduate-entry medicine courses and their required admissions test

University	Pre-admissions test
Bangor	UCAT
Cambridge	None
Cardiff	UCAT
Chester	UCAT
King's	UCAT
Newcastle	UCAT
Nottingham	GAMSAT
Oxford	To be decided
Queen Mary	UCAT
ScotGEM	GAMSAT
Sheffield	UCAT
Southampton	UCAT
St George's	GAMSAT
Surrey	UCAT or GAMSAT
Swansea	GAMSAT
Ulster	GAMSAT
Warwick	UCAT
Worcester	UCAT or GAMSAT

Standard registrations for the GAMSAT UK test take place in May for those sitting the test in September, and in November for those sitting the test in March. The fee to sit the GAMSAT test is £271, but an extra charge of £65 applies if you register for the GAMSAT after the main closing date. Payment must be made at the time of completing your online registration. Candidates sit the GAMSAT examination in either March or September, and those with the best all-round scores are then called for interview. The GAMSAT examination consists of three papers, which are all taken on the same day.

1. Reasoning in humanities and social sciences (62 multiple-choice questions) – 100 minutes, including 8 minutes' reading time.
2. Written communication (two writing tasks) – 65 minutes, including 5 minutes' reading time.
3. Reasoning in biological and physical sciences (75 multiple-choice questions: 40% biology, 40% chemistry, 20% physics) – 150 minutes, including 8 minutes' reading time.

The GAMSAT website (https://gamsat.acer.org) contains full details of the test along with practice test materials. This is a far more significant test than the UCAT and, as such, it would be expected that more time is spent in preparation for it.

Private universities

At the University of Buckingham, the first private medical school in the UK opened in January 2015. It currently costs £40,000 per year for a home student and £45,000 for an international student, and will fast-track medical students in four-and-a-half years rather than the standard five or six years. The university is hoping to attract students who would otherwise have looked to study abroad and, as such, is potentially of interest to mature students.

Studying outside the UK

If you are unsuccessful in gaining a place at a UK medical school, and do not want to follow the graduate-entry path, there are other options.

One option for those who have been unsuccessful with their applications is to study medicine abroad – for example at Charles University in the Czech Republic or Comenius University in Bratislava, the capital of Slovakia. There are a number of medical schools throughout the world that will accept A level students, but the important issue is whether or not you would be able to practise in the UK upon qualification, should you wish to do so. You need to bear in mind that there is a big difference between European and non-European medical schools. In the case of medical schools based within the EU, they are usually fully recognised by the GMC under current European legislation for primary qualifications.

Note that following the UK's decision to leave the EU, arrangements for UK students studying at institutions in other EU countries have changed. If you wish to study a whole degree course in an EU member state, it is likely that you will pay a different level of fees which will be based on international student fees.

It is important to be cautious when considering studying abroad outside of the EU, as differences in culture, teaching styles and university life in general can be something of a shock. Make sure you carry out extensive research into prospective universities, and be cautious in your approach.

There are a wide range of courses outside of the EU attended by UK students. To then practise in the UK, students must sit the PLAB (Professional and Linguistic Assessment Board) test before applying for registration (www.gmc-uk.org/registration-and-licensing/join-the-register/plab). An example of a well-known non-EU course is St George's

University School of Medicine in Grenada. Students who wish to practise in the UK can spend part of the clinical stage of the course in a range of hospitals in the UK. Clinical experience can also be gained in hospitals in the US, allowing students to practise there as well. A high proportion of the St George's University medical school teachers have worked in UK universities and medical schools.

In order to check if your qualification is recognised in the UK, you should visit the GMC website (www.gmc-uk.org/registration-and-licensing/join-the-register/before-you-apply/acceptable-overseas-qualifications). You can also refer to the university websites, which should inform you of the validity of their degree in the UK.

Studying abroad may not be the first choice for students who were initially hoping to secure a place at home in the UK. Also, healthcare systems outside the UK are very different, so adapting to life abroad where the local language may not be English as well as studying medicine may not appeal to all.

Case study

After completing her A levels in the UK, Shifa opted to undertake her studies at the University of Constanta in Romania. She recently completed her degree and has since returned to the UK to start working as a doctor. She is particularly interested in working in oncology, haematology, radiology and pathology at this early stage in her career.

'The most rewarding thing about a healthcare career is the ability to make a positive difference in the lives of patients and the community, – along with medicine's intellectual, emotional, and moral fulfilment.

'The life of a doctor is often romanticised as a noble and rewarding profession, and rightfully so. However, beneath the white coats and stethoscopes lie these dedicated individuals facing daily tough challenges. The challenges of being a doctor include coping with long and unpredictable work hours, emotional distress from witnessing suffering and loss, high levels of stress from exams, the struggle to maintain a work–life balance, significant financial pressures, the need for continuous learning and adaptation to evolving medical technology, and the challenges of working within complex healthcare team dynamics. Breaking bad news is something I found initially very challenging. When these challenges are faced and overcome, it provides excellent job satisfaction, making the medical profession both demanding and rewarding.

'In terms of things that are current in the practice of medicine, it is worth remembering that we are the first generation of doctors to be working with AI (Artificial Intelligence). There is a current rise in digital health through telemedicine, wearable devices, and health apps; it offers timely and convenient access to medical services, empowers individuals to manage their health proactively, facilitates the collection and analysis of vast patient data for more precise treatments, and ultimately strives to make healthcare more efficient, personalised, and globally accessible. Something interesting is the use of digital stethoscopes – these are modern versions of traditional acoustic stethoscopes, which incorporate digital technology to enhance how medical professionals listen to and analyse heart and lung sounds.

'Another thing I find incredible is that we are now doing surgeries with the assistance of robots. Surgeons control these robotic systems and provide highly detailed movements, reducing the margin of error in delicate procedures. AI algorithms also assist surgeons by providing real-time data analysis, image processing and predictive insights, allowing for better decision-making during surgery. Integrating robots and AI in surgery offers a promising future for minimally invasive, highly accurate, and efficient procedures, with potential benefits in reduced pain, faster recovery and improved patient safety.

'My key advice for anyone aspiring to be a medic is that you must be passionate and motivated. It is not an easy profession, and it is a lifelong commitment to studying and adapting. Do as much work experience as you can. Prioritise your physical and mental well-being, and balance your professional and personal life. You must be dedicated to your job to be a great doctor and enjoy your work.'

Getting into US medical schools

While it is possible for international students to study medicine in the United States, it certainly is not straightforward. Firstly, you should go to the AAMC (Association of American Medical Colleges) website at www.aamc.org. This is an excellent site, but can be difficult to navigate to find the information you need. All of the member universities are listed, and by following the links most of your questions can be answered.

Furthermore, from here you can be directed to AMCAS, which is the American Medical College Application Service. For students wishing to apply, go to https://students-residents.aamc.org. The fee is $175 for an application to one school and $45 for every school applied to thereafter. The AAMC website suggests that a very good investment is the *Medical School Admission Requirements* (MSAR), which can be bought as an online resource from https://students-residents.aamc.org/medical-school-admission-requirements/medical-school-admission-requirements-msar-applicants.

In the US, medicine is a postgraduate degree. All medical students have completed four years of a science-based or pre-med undergraduate course. You are also expected to gain work experience in the first two years. For more information go to https://students-residents.aamc.org/aspiring-docs/aspiring-docs.

Suffice to say that the following criteria have to be met.

- Very high grades in A levels – nearly all straight A grades. The higher the grades, the higher your GPA (grade point average) will be; the higher your GPA, the better your chances of being selected by the more renowned universities. An A grade = 4 GPA points; a B grade = 3 points; and a C = 2 points.
- At least one year of biology, physics and English and two years of chemistry (including organic chemistry) post-16/at A level.
- A first degree in a science subject.
- Two or three references from your personal tutor and teachers.
- If you are not from an English-speaking country you may be required to sit the TOEFL (Test of English as a Foreign Language). The minimum score for entry into any university is 80 out of 120. The more demanding the course (such as medicine) and the more prestigious the university, the higher this language requirement will be. Most universities also accept the IELTS (International English Language Testing System). The TOEFL test and the IELTS can be sat in the UK.

If you are serious about applying, you need to start as early as possible – early in the first year of your undergraduate programme is recommended. This is because you will need to research the universities as best you can, bearing in mind that the distance does not allow for quick visits to open days as for UK universities. It is also important to remember that fees and living costs are very high; a list of fees and costs can be obtained from the AAMC website.

MCAT

Almost every medical school in the US and Canada requires students to take this 7.5-hour examination administered by AAMC. It is a computer-based, multiple-choice assessment, which is divided into four sections.

1. Biological and Biochemical Foundations of Living Systems.
2. Chemical and Physical Foundations of Biological Systems.
3. Psychological, Social, and Biological Foundations of Behaviour.
4. Critical Analysis and Reasoning Skills.

This exam is to be taken in the year that you intend to start study. You can take it up to three times in a year, or four times over two years and a maximum of seven times in your lifetime. Test dates tend to generally be spread between January and September each year, and you are recommended to register at least 60 days beforehand to ensure that you get a place. It costs $335.

Visas

If you are studying abroad, you will usually require a visa for study. Following the withdrawal of the UK from the European Union, the rules for UK students studying in Europe have changed, so you will need to check carefully what the requirements are. A good place to start this research is www.gov.uk/guidance/study-in-the-european-union#doing-your-whole-course-at-a-higher-education-provider-in-the-eu.

For studying in the USA, the university in question will best advise you on which visa you should obtain; for example, they will advise you as to whether you require an F-1 Student visa. You do not require a student visa for Grenada if you have a valid British passport. A good place to look first would be the website for the US embassy in the UK at https://uk.usembassy.gov/visas/study-exchange/student.

Students with disabilities and special educational needs

If a candidate has a specific health requirement or disability there is every possibility that a medical school will be able to help. There is an area in the personal details section of the UCAS application where you can indicate the type of disability/special needs that you have. You need to select the most appropriate option from the list given. There is also a space provided for you to give any further details of the conditions that affect you.

However, each medical school has a responsibility to ensure that doctors are able to fulfil their responsibilities. The decision on fitness to practise is separate from the academic and non-academic selection process. These guidelines are set out by the GMC. You are encouraged to fully research the demands of the course before you apply to each institution. The profession places huge demands on the individual and therefore you must consider all the facts from the outset.

You are equally encouraged to apply if you have a hearing or visual impairment. All institutions are fully committed to support students with special needs, from dyslexia to physical disability, and have access arrangements in place.

Once an offer is made, the medical school will contact you to discuss any appropriate arrangements that should be made. It is absolutely vital that all relevant information that may impair your ability to study and potentially practise is made clear at this stage. If not, and if the issues become obvious later on in the course, it could possibly result in the candidate being withdrawn from the course.

In terms of special educational needs, students who require a word processor or extra time will be allowed these in the same way that they would have been at school, subject to providing the correct documentation to the university. For more information refer directly to the university.

Some useful websites

Health Careers: www.healthcareers.nhs.uk/career-planning/study-and-training/considering-or-university/support-university/disability-support
GMC: www.gmc-uk.org/education/standards-guidance-and-curricula/guidance/welcomed-and-valued/health-and-disability-in-medicine

10 | Fees and funding

Whether undertaking an undergraduate or postgraduate course, the cost of studying is considerable. This has been exacerbated in recent years by rises in living costs due to inflation alongside the cost of university tuition fees. A study released by the British Medical Association in 2022 (www.bma.org.uk/media/6069/bma-student-survey-2022.pdf) calculated that average debt among medical students in England was £54,342, with values ranging from £600 to £210,500.

When considering levels of student debt, it is easy to become disheartened and think that university study is not for you. What all students must remember is that tuition fees do not have to be paid up front; in fact, most students receive student loans to cover this cost. In addition, the loans do not start to be paid back until you are earning over a certain amount (see page 190). However, it can be a real challenge for many students to pay for living costs, such as rent and food, so it is vital to be aware of how you will meet these expenses.

Undertaking a course such as medicine should only be done after seriously considering the overall cost and carefully examining your ability to be fully committed to your study for the full five years. Try to plan your finances in advance so that you are prepared to cover the cost of tuition fees, living expenses, books and other necessary equipment. Remember, living costs in big cities such as London will be much higher than in other parts of the country.

To find out what the fees are and what funding is available for medical courses, you should explore each of the universities' websites, because fees and funding procedures vary from university to university. However, due to the high quality of education provided by medical schools, it is usual for them to charge the maximum level of fees permitted.

Fees

UK students

The tuition fee that you will have to pay for undergraduate courses will depend on where you live and where you intend to study. Universities are allowed to charge Home undergraduate fees up to £9,250 per year, as part of the government's Teaching Excellence Framework (TEF), which assesses universities and colleges on the quality of their teaching. The fee cap for students studying in Wales remains at £9,000, while fees for students in Northern Ireland are a maximum of £9,250 for 2024 entry. These fees have been the same for a number of years and have been frozen until at least the 2024/2025 academic year, but increases are expected in the future.

There are a number of variations between the systems in England, Scotland, Wales and Northern Ireland, which can result in significant differences between the fees that are ultimately paid by students. Currently (for 2023/2024 entry) the rules are as follows, although they may be subject to change in the future.

- Students from England are required to pay a maximum of £9,250 if they are studying in England, Scotland or Northern Ireland, and up to £9,000 if they are studying in Wales.
- Students from Scotland who study at Scottish universities are not required to pay tuition fees (or, rather, tuition fees of £1,820 for 2024 entry are covered the Student Awards Agency for Scotland (SAAS) for students who qualify for home student status). Scottish students have to pay fees of up to £9,250 if they study in England or Northern Ireland, and up to £9,000 if they study in Wales.
- Students from Wales pay up to £9,000 if they study in Wales, or up to £9,250 if they study in England, Scotland or Northern Ireland.
- Students living in Northern Ireland pay up to £4,710 if they attend university in Northern Ireland, up to £9,250 if they study in England or Scotland, and up to £9,000 if they study in Wales.

EU and non-EU international students

At present, EU students are charged the same fees as non-EU international students, which are significantly higher than those charged to UK students and are determined by each university. Some students from the EU may be eligible for some support in terms of student loans from the UK government, but this is dependent on a number of factors, so it is best to check personal eligibility. Students from the Republic of Ireland are exempt from paying higher fees and are eligible for home fee status.

Living expenses

Your living expenses include the cost of your accommodation, food, clothes, travel and equipment, leisure and social activities – plus possible extras like field trips and study visits, if these aren't covered by the tuition fees.

Check university and college websites for information about possible living costs. Some offer more detailed advice than others, and give breakdowns under various headings such as accommodation, food and daily travel. Others go even further and give typical weekly, monthly or annual spends.

If you're living away from home, accommodation will make up the largest proportion of your living costs. There is likely to be a range of accommodation options – from a standard room in university halls through to privately rented accommodation – with a range of price points. You'll probably be surprised when you do some research to find that the cheapest and most expensive towns are not as you might have expected; the cost of accommodation often depends on how much of it is available in a particular area.

When choosing accommodation, it is essential to consider its location and factor in the cost of travel to your university or college. It is also important to find out what's included in the accommodation costs (such as utilities, personal property insurance and Wi-Fi) and whether it is possible to pay for accommodation during term time only.

Funding your studies

How do you fund your time in higher education? Don't ignore this question and leave it until the last minute! You will need to think carefully about how to budget for several years' costs – and you need to know what help you might get from:

- the government
- your family or partner
- paid part-time work
- other sources, such as bursaries and scholarships.

This chapter gives a brief overview of a complicated funding situation, which can vary according to where you come from and where you plan to study. For more details about the different types of funding available and how to apply for them, check your regional student finance website.

- **England:** www.gov.uk/student-finance.
- **Wales:** www.studentfinancewales.co.uk.
- **Scotland:** www.saas.gov.uk.
- **Northern Ireland:** www.studentfinanceni.co.uk.

Tuition fee loans

For UK students, tuition fees can be covered by taking out a tuition fee loan, which will be paid directly to your university or college at the start of each year of your course. You are effectively given a loan by the government that you repay through your income tax from the April after you finish your course but only once your earnings reach a certain threshold. Currently, these income thresholds stand at:

- £25,000 per year for students from England
- £27,295 per year for students from Wales
- £27,660 per year for students from Scotland (who go to university outside of Scotland)
- £22,015 per year for students from Northern Ireland.

(All figures apply to students starting their course after 1 August 2023.)

So, if you never reach this threshold, you will not have to repay the fees. In addition, any outstanding balance on your loan will be cancelled after a certain period of time if you have not already cleared it in full. The length of time depends on the rules at the time you took out the loan. For students from England who started their studies in September 2023, the repayment period was recently extended to 40 years (from 30 years), so it is recommended that students in other regions keep a close eye on any developments with respect to the length of the loan repayment period.

The current situation regarding repayments is that you repay 9% of anything you earn over the annual income threshold.

The interest rate charged on student loans depends on what repayment plan you are on, but for students in England who started their course after 1 August 2023 (Plan 5) it is set at the RPI (Retail Price Index) rate of inflation.

Maintenance loans

In addition to a tuition fee loan, all students can apply for a maintenance or living cost loan; however, the amount you can borrow will be dependent on your household income – in other words, it is means tested. 'Household income' refers to your family's gross annual income (their income before tax). With the exception of loans available to Scottish students, the amount you can claim also varies depending on your living situation, with the maximum loan being available to students living away from home in London.

Each regional student finance website includes a finance calculator tool that will give an estimate of the finance you would be eligible for based on your family income and other factors, and it is well worth looking at this before planning your budget.

England (2024/25)

The maximum annual maintenance loan in England:

- £8,610 for those living in the family home
- £10,227 for those living away from home (£13,348 in London).

Wales (2023/24)

In Wales, students can get a combination of a maintenance grant, which they do not have to pay back, and a maintenance loan. Although the grants are means tested, most students will get a grant of at least £1,000.

The maximum amounts for maintenance loans and grants in Wales:

- £9,950 for those living in the family home
- £11,720 for those living away from home (£14,365 in London).

Scotland (2024/25)

In Scotland, students can get a mix of maintenance loans and non-repayable bursaries (grants) to cover living expenses. These are as follows (all figures per year):

- household income up to £20,999: £2,000 bursary and £9,400 loan
- household income £21,000–£23,999: £1,125 bursary and £9,400 loan
- household income £24,000–£33,999: £500 bursary and £9,400 loan
- household income £34,000 and above: no bursary and £8,400 loan.

Unlike the rest of the UK, bursaries and loan eligibility for Scottish students is calculated using the income bands listed above rather than exact household income.

Northern Ireland (2023/24)

The maximum annual maintenance loan in Northern Ireland:

- £5,250 for those living in the family home
- £6,776 for those living away from home (£9,492 in London).

In addition, you may be eligible for a non-repayable maintenance grant if your household income is below £41,065. This is paid alongside any maintenance loan you qualify for and is up to £3,475.

Additional support

Bursaries and scholarships

What's the difference? Bursaries are usually non-competitive and automatic, often based on financial need, while scholarships are competitive and you usually have to apply for them. However, many universities and colleges use the terms interchangeably.

NHS bursaries

Currently, students studying for medical degrees recognised by the General Medical Council may be eligible for financial assistance from the NHS for part of their course. The arrangements vary depending on your country of residence, and are set out briefly below.

England

For qualifying students, tuition fees are paid by the NHS Student Bursary scheme from the fifth year of study onwards. They will also be able to apply for a means-tested NHS bursary for living costs of up to £2,643 per year (outside London if not living with parents). The bursary award also includes access to a non-means-tested grant of £1,000.

Wales

For qualifying students, tuition fees are paid in the fifth year and students can apply for a means-tested NHS Bursary (administered by Student Awards Services) from the fifth year of their course of up to £2,643 per year. Students also receive a non-means-tested grant of £1,000.

Scotland

For qualifying students, tuition fees for those studying in Scotland are paid by the Student Awards Agency Scotland (SAAS) for the duration of the course. Students can apply to the SAAS for maintenance support, which includes loans and bursaries throughout the course.

Northern Ireland

For qualifying students, income-assessed bursaries are available from the fifth year onwards. The bursaries are administered by the Department of Health, and tuition fees are also paid by the Department for the duration of the bursary. While in receipt of the bursary, students can also apply for a reduced maintenance loan from Student Finance Northern Ireland.

Further details and guidelines are available on the NHS Business Services Authority website at www.nhsbsa.nhs.uk/nhs-bursary-students.

Other sources of funding for medical students

There are various websites that will give you information on a variety of organisations that can offer scholarships, grants and bursaries that are available in addition to the NHS bursary. These include the following.

- **Armed forces bursaries/cadetships:** these are generous and may be worth considering, provided you are happy to commit to an agreed number of years working as a doctor in the Army, Navy or Air Force.
- **University bursaries:** some universities often provide bursaries for low-income students; some also give bursaries to people with higher incomes. The arrangements in place at each university differ, so it is worth investigating this directly with them.
- **Hardship funds:** if you are having financial problems you can apply for additional sources of funding from your institution. This is usually in the form of a bursary that doesn't have to be repaid, but might

take the form of a loan. Hardship funds are administered individually by each university, so it is best to discuss directly with them.
- Students with children or responsibility for dependent adults can apply for a range of support including Childcare Grant, Parents' Learning Allowance and Child Tax Credit.
- Disabled students can apply for Disabled Students' Allowance.
- Organisations such as the Royal Medical Benevolent Fund (RMBF) (https://rmbf.org) can offer means-tested grants to individuals facing financial hardship due to ill health, disability or bereavement.

For more information on these, go to www.gov.uk/student-finance/extra-help and the individual university websites.

Scholarships and prizes

There are also many scholarships and prizes that are run by the many professional medical organisations. Some of the applications may require a supporting statement from a member of academic staff. Check the criteria carefully before applying.

- **British Association of Dermatologists:** offers a range of bursaries, fellowships and awards to students and professionals at different stages of their careers. Visit www.bad.org.uk/education-training/bursaries-fellowships-awards for more details.
- **Sir John Ellis Student Prizes:** students submit a description of a piece of work, survey, research or innovation in which they have been directly involved in the field of medical education. Each category awards a monetary prize and the opportunity to present their work. Visit www.asme.org.uk for more details.
- **The Genetics Society Summer Studentship scheme:** this provides funding for undergraduate students to spend their summer vacation working in a genetics laboratory in order to gain research experience: £300 per week for up to eight weeks and £750 to contribute to costs incurred in the lab work. There are different grants available to cover any course-specific costs. Visit https://genetics.org.uk/grants/summer-studentships for more details.
- **The Physiological Society:** the Society offers a range of grants for students undertaking research of a physiologic nature under the supervision of a member of the Society during a summer vacation or intercalated BSc year (if the student is not receiving LA or other government support). Visit www.physoc.org/grants-and-prizes/grants for more details.
- **The Pathological Society:** funding is offered for students wanting to intercalate a BSc in pathology who do not have LA or other government support. The Society also offers awards to fund electives and vacation studies in pathology. Visit www.pathsoc.org/grants_lectures_awards/default.aspx for more details.

Websites such as The Scholarship Hub (www.thescholarshiphub.org.uk) can also be a useful resource for finding details of available funding.

Fees for studying abroad

You should not expect the same level of financial support if you want to study overseas. If you move to the EU to start a course, you will need to pay different fee rates compared to before Brexit. It is worth visiting individual university websites to find out the cost of studying there.

You can find out more about financial support for studying in the EU at www.gov.uk/guidance/study-in-the-european-union#doing-your-whole-course-at-a-higher-education-provider-in-the-eu.

Case study

Deterred by the competition to study medicine in the UK, Usmaan conducted research into studying abroad. Usmaan is now is his fourth year, studying at Constanta in Romania.

'From a young age I was fascinated by medicine. The combination of ethics and science motivated me to pursue medicine as a career, as well as my interest in human anatomy. With all these things in mind, I did a lot of research into the course and undertook various work experience placements, which further fuelled my passion for studying medicine.

'We all know that getting a medical school place in the UK is difficult because it is so competitive, even if you have secured outstanding grades. I was determined that medicine was the right course for me and I didn't want to settle for anything less. My sister was already studying abroad, so I was familiar with the possibility of doing so, as well as the application process and realities of studying in a different country.

'As with anything in life, studying medicine abroad has its pros and cons. That being said, I definitely feel that I made the right choice. Being far away from home makes you more independent, stronger and equips you with invaluable skills for medicine and life in general. To begin with it was hard – give yourself time to settle in and find your feet – but I quickly made friends and got into the study routine. The majority of students and staff speak English and there are many restaurants, bars and gyms to spend your leisure time. You have the option to travel home during the holidays, but social media means that it is easier than ever to stay in touch with your friends and family back home. There are many British people on the course, but it has also been great to socialise with people from lots of different backgrounds.

'The application process was fairly simple as I applied through an agent who handled most of the paperwork for me. Once my paperwork had been approved, I had to sit an entrance exam which was difficult, but a couple of months before the exam, the university provided me with practice material to get an idea of what the exam would be like. Once I had passed the exam, I received an acceptance letter confirming my place at the university, which allowed me to enrol. The agent also helped me to find an apartment, set up a new phone and gave me a tour around the area to familiarise me with it.

'Before applying to study medicine, I undertook work experience at a range of places, in charity shops, retail, pharmacies and hospitals. It's important to undertake placements in a range of areas to ensure that medicine is the right path for you. It also helped me to develop social skills, and this is important when dealing with patients further down the line and when working in a team.

'I would say my path into medicine was an unusual one as it took me longer than usual to get a place. This was purely down to my lack of commitment early on, my work ethic and my self-belief. However, I had a lot of support from my tutors at college who helped me to stay on track and pushed me to achieve the grades I needed when I was retaking my A levels, which allowed me to secure the A and A* grades I needed. My teachers were really proactive and if there was an area I was lacking in, they would pick up on this and push me in the right direction.

'Studying medicine has its ups and downs, but overall it has been a very good course. It is not easy because of the sheer amount of content, but once you get into a good study routine, managing this gets easier. For the first two years, I really enjoyed anatomy which is the foundation of any medical student's knowledge. From third year onwards, everything is clinical based, and I am in the hospital every day, putting my theoretical knowledge into practice. Once clinical placements start, you feel more like a doctor, which is particularly enjoyable. I have particularly enjoyed my orthopaedics rotation so far. Covid-19 has restricted our clinical practice to a degree, but it has been interesting to study in this context.

'In the long run, I would like to become a consultant, but I am not sure which field I would like to specialise in just yet, as I am still to experience many more, including dermatology and gynaecology.

'I would advise prospective medical students not to lose focus. You might feel like giving up at times, but you have to persevere, especially when you are completing your A levels and everything is up in the air. You should keep the end result in the back of your mind and by taking each day as you come, you can slowly but surely work towards your goals.'

11 | Careers in medicine

This chapter looks briefly at some of the possible careers open to prospective medics. It is of value to understand some of the avenues open to you after graduation, even if you have no firm idea about which one you want to pursue at this point.

The paths and avenues open to members of the medical profession once they graduate are too numerous to go into in detail here. As a trainee doctor nearing the end of your study, questions such as the prospect and possibility of specialisation and about where you might like to work have to be answered. The best advice we can give here is to make sure to research as much as possible, talk to people and, above all, be aware of the areas in medicine that you have enjoyed the most.

Apart from specialisations (see below), there is a wide range of areas that doctors may end up working in. Most people understand that many doctors become GPs or work in hospitals. However, there are also as many who dedicate their lives to working in areas such as public health, medical management and administration, and research.

Away from hospitals, there are careers to be made in private enterprise, for example running a consultancy business such as plastic surgery. Some doctors opt for the armed forces and others work for the police as forensic psychiatrists and forensic pathologists. Another area is education, in terms of lecturing, research and writing while working for a university. It is not uncommon to find doctors who have a portfolio of work, spending some of their time in hospitals, doing private consultancy in their own surgeries and teaching or doing research. Such a life is not only well remunerated but also highly stimulating.

First job

The training programme for doctors called Modernising Medical Careers (MMC) became fully functional in 2007. The training ultimately leads to the awarding of the Foundation Programme Certificate of Completion (FPCC). MMC is summarised in Figure 4 (see page 198).

In the last year of the medical degree, medical students apply for a place on the Foundation programme and then gain provisional GMC registration once the last year is completed. The Foundation programme is designed to provide structured postgraduate training on the job and lasts two years. The job starts a few weeks after graduation from medical school. In the first few weeks there might be a short period of 'shadowing', to help new doctors get used to the job. After successful completion of the first year, they will gain registration with the GMC.

The Foundation programme job is divided into three four-month posts in the first year. These posts will typically consist of:

- four months of surgery (e.g. urology, general surgery)
- four months of another specialty (e.g. psychiatry, general practice)
- four months in a medical specialty (e.g. respiratory, geriatrics).

The second year is again divided into three four-month posts, but here the focus is perhaps on a specialty or may include other jobs in shortage areas.

Final year at medical school: apply for a place on a two-year Foundation programme (www.foundationprogramme.nhs.uk)

↓

Foundation programme starts in August
F1: three four-month placements (medicine, surgery, specialty)
F2: three four-month placements (some choice of placements)
During F2, apply for General Practice vocational training programme or other specialty

↓

Specialty training begins
GP registrar: approximately three years
Other specialty: five to eight years
After completion, receive Foundation Programme Certificate of Completion (FPCC)

↓

Apply for senior posts, e.g. consultant

Figure 4 MMC training structure

For more information on the application procedure, visit:

- www.foundationprogramme.nhs.uk
- www.healthcareers.nhs.uk/explore-roles/doctors

Specialisations

Specialist training programmes typically last three years for general practice, and five to eight years for other specialities. After gaining the FPCC (or Certificate of Eligibility for Specialist Registration (CESR) if you trained abroad), you will be eligible for entry to the GMC's Specialist Register or GP Register.

To do this you will need to apply for postgraduate medical training programmes in the UK to the deanery or 'unit of application' directly. In this application process you will be competing for places on specialty training programmes with other doctors at similar levels of competence and experience.

For more information, visit NHS Health Education England at https://medical.hee.nhs.uk/medical-training-recruitment.

Below are the major specialisations available in medicine.

- Acute Medicine
- ACCS (Acute Care Common Stem) Emergency Medicine
- Allergy
- Anaesthetics
- Anaesthetics and ACCS Anaesthetics
- Audiovestibular Medicine
- Cardiology
- Cardiothoracic Surgery
- Child and Adolescent Psychiatry
- Clinical Genetics
- Clinical Neurophysiology
- Clinical Oncology
- Clinical Pharmacology and Therapeutics
- Clinical Radiology
- Combined Infection Training
- Community Sexual and Reproductive Health
- Core Psychiatry Training
- Core Surgical Training
- Dermatology
- Diagnostic Neuropathology
- Emergency Medicine – Direct Route of Entry
- Emergency Medicine
- Endocrinology and Diabetes
- Gastroenterology
- General Practice
- General Surgery and Vascular Surgery
- Genito-urinary Medicine
- Geriatric Medicine
- Haematology
- Histopathology
- Immunology
- Intensive Care Medicine
- Internal Medicine Training and ACCS Acute Medicine
- Medical Oncology
- Medical Ophthalmology
- Metabolic Medicine
- Neurology
- Neurosurgery
- Nuclear Medicine
- Obstetrics and Gynaecology
- Occupational Medicine
- Ophthalmology
- Oral and Maxillofacial Surgery
- Otolaryngology (Ears, Nose and Throat)
- Paediatric and Perinatal Pathology
- Paediatric Cardiology
- Paediatric Surgery
- Paediatrics
- Palliative Medicine
- Plastic Surgery
- Public Health
- Rehabilitation Medicine
- Renal Medicine
- Respiratory Medicine
- Rheumatology
- Sports and Exercise Medicine
- Trauma and Orthopaedic Surgery
- Urology

A few selected specialisations, briefly described, follow.

Anaesthetist

An anaesthetist is a medical doctor trained to administer anaesthesia and manage the medical care of patients before, during and after surgery. Anaesthetists are the single largest group of hospital doctors and their skills are used throughout the hospital in patient care. They have a medical background to deal with many emergency situations. They are also trained to deal with breathing, resuscitation of the heart and lungs and advanced life support.

Audiologist

Audiologists identify and assess hearing and/or balance disorders, and from this will recommend and provide appropriate rehabilitation for the patient. The main areas of work are paediatrics, adult assessment and rehabilitation, special needs groups and research and development.

Cardiologist

This is the branch of medicine that deals with disorders of the heart and blood vessels. These specialists deal with the diagnosis and treatment of heart defects, heart failure and valvular heart disease.

Dermatologist

There are over 2,000 recognised diseases of the skin but about 20 of these account for 90% of the workload. Dermatologists diagnose and treat diseases of the skin, hair and nails such as severe acne in teenagers, which is a very common reason for referral. Inflammatory skin diseases such as eczema and psoriasis are also common and without treatment can produce significant disability.

Emergency

Often referred to as the type of medicine practised in accident and emergency departments. It requires doctors to be dynamic and ready to adapt and respond at a moment's notice. Departments are led by consultants but rely on teamwork to help patients who are in an urgent condition. As you might be required to make life-saving decisions in a pressurised situation you will need a lot of confidence and belief to be in this role.

Gastroenterologist

A gastroenterologist is a medically qualified specialist who has sub-specialised in the diseases of the digestive system, which include ailments affecting all organs, from mouth to anus, along the alimentary canal. In all, a gastroenterologist undergoes a minimum of 13 years of formal classroom education and practical training before becoming a gastroenterologist.

General practitioner (GP)

A GP is a medical practitioner who specialises in family medicine and primary care. They are often referred to as family doctors and work in consultation clinics based in the local community.

GPs can work on their own or in a group practice with other doctors and healthcare providers. A GP treats acute and chronic illnesses and provides care and health education for all ages. They are called GPs because they look after a whole person, and this includes their mental health and physical well-being.

Gynaecologist

Gynaecologists have a broad base of knowledge and can vary their professional focus on different disorders and diseases of the female reproductive system. This includes preventive care, prenatal care and detection of sexually transmitted diseases, smear-test screening and family planning. They may choose to specialise in different areas, such as acute and chronic medical conditions, for example cervical cancer, infertility, urinary tract disorders and pregnancy and delivery.

Immunologist

Immunologists are responsible for investigating the functions of the body's immune system. They help to treat diseases such as AIDS/HIV, allergies (e.g. asthma, hay fever) and leukaemia using complex and sophisticated molecular techniques. They deal with the understanding of the processes and effects of inappropriate stimulation that are associated with allergies and transplant rejection, and may be heavily involved with research. An immunologist works within clinical and academic settings as well as with industrial research. Their role involves measuring components of the immune system, including cells, antibodies and other proteins. They develop new therapies, which involves looking at how to improve methods for treating different conditions.

Neurologist

A neurologist is trained in the diagnosis and treatment of nervous-system disorders, which includes diseases of the brain, spinal cord, nerves and muscles. They perform medical examinations of the nerves of the head and neck, muscle strength and movement, balance, ambulation and reflexes, memory, speech, language and other cognitive abilities.

Obstetrician

These are specialised doctors who deal with problems that arise during maternity care, treating any complications that develop in pregnancy and childbirth and any that arise after the birth. Some obstetricians may specialise in a particular aspect of maternity care such as maternal medicine, which involves looking after the mother's health; labour care, which involves care during the birth; and/or foetal medicine, which involves looking after the health of the unborn baby.

Paediatrician

Paediatricians deal with the growth, development and health of children from birth to adolescence. To become paediatricians, doctors must complete six years of extra training after they finish their medical training. There are general paediatricians and specialist paediatricians such as paediatric cardiologists. They work in private practices or hospitals.

Plastic surgeon

Plastic surgery is the medical and cosmetic specialty that involves the correction of form and function. There are two main types of plastic surgery: cosmetic and reconstructive.

1. Cosmetic surgery procedures alter a part of the body that the person is not satisfied with.
2. Reconstructive plastic surgery involves correcting physical birth defects, such as cleft palates, or defects that occur as a result of disease treatments, such as breast reconstruction after a mastectomy, or from accidents, such as third-degree burns after a fire.

Plastic surgery includes a variety of fields such as hand surgery, burn surgery, microsurgery and paediatric surgery.

Psychiatrist

Psychiatrists are trained in the medical, psychological and social components of mental, emotional and behavioural disorders. They specialise in the prevention, diagnosis and treatment of mental, addictive and emotional disorders such as anxiety, depression, psychosis, substance abuse and developmental disabilities. They prescribe medications, practise psychotherapy and help patients and their families cope with stress and crises. Psychiatrists often consult with primary care physicians, psychotherapists, psychologists and social workers.

Surgeon

A general surgeon is a physician who has been educated and trained in diagnosis, operative and post-operative treatment, and management of patient care. Surgery requires extensive knowledge of anatomy, emergency and intensive care, nutrition, pathology, shock and resuscitation, and wound healing. Surgeons may practise in specific fields such as general surgery, orthopaedic, neurological or vascular and many more.

Urologist

A urologist is a physician who has specialised knowledge and skills regarding problems of the male and female urinary tracts and the male reproductive organs. Extensive knowledge of internal medicine, paediatrics, gynaecology and other specialties is required by the urologist.

Some alternative careers

Army

Doctors in the Army are also officers, and provide medical care for soldiers and their families (https://jobs.army.mod.uk/roles/army-medical-service/doctor).

Aviation medicine (also aerospace medicine)

The main role is to assess the fitness to fly of pilots, cabin crew and infirm passengers (for further information go to the website of the Faculty of Occupational Medicine www.fom.ac.uk).

Clinical forensic medical examiner (police surgeon)

Clinical forensic physicians or medical examiners spend much of their time examining people who have been arrested. Detainees either ask to see a doctor or need to be examined to see if they are fit for interview or fit to be detained (www.csofs.org).

Coroner

The coroner is responsible for inquiring into violent, sudden and unexpected, unnatural or suspicious deaths. Few are doctors, but some have qualifications in both medicine and law.

Pathologist

This job requires a variety of different specialisms, all of which combine to help form the basis of medical diagnosis. Whether it be chemical pathology, haematology, histopathology or immunology, each of which then breaks down further, there is a variety of opportunities available in clinical and lab-based research work.

Pharmaceutical medicine

Job opportunities for doctors in pharmaceutical medicine include clinical research, medical advisory positions and becoming the medical director of a company. Patient contact is limited but still possible in the clinical trials area (www.abpi.org.uk).

Prison medicine

A prison medical officer provides healthcare, usually in the form of GP clinics, to prison inmates.

Public health practitioner

Public health medicine is a specialty that deals with health at the level of a general population rather than at the level of the individual. The role can vary from responding to outbreaks of disease that need a rapid response, such as food poisoning, to the long-term planning of health-care (www.fph.org.uk).

> *'What is special about medicine? Everything and nothing. Everything because you have the ability to help and make a difference to people's lives. Nothing, because once you go into this career, it is your duty and part of your everyday routine. What you do matters but it is also expected. You must be serious about what you want to do because there will be many relying on you. It is tremendously rewarding and that is why anyone should go to work. In regards to the application, simply be true to you; that is the best starting place.'*
>
> *Dr Emma Lumley*

12 | Further information

Courses

Students often have a variety of reasons for wanting to dedicate their professional lives to medicine. However, each aspiring 'future doctor' must ensure that this career choice has been an informed one. It is impossible to get a true idea of what medicine entails from just attending a course or talking to careers advisers. However, there are a number of organisations that aim to help students gain a realistic impression of medicine as a whole. Medic Mentor (https://medicmentor.co.uk) is one such organisation that provides useful courses and resources for prospective medical students.

Publications

Careers in medicine

Being Mortal, Atul Gawande, Profile Books

Breaking & Mending: A Junior Doctor's Stories of Compassion & Burn-out, Joanna Cannon, Wellcome Collection

This is Going to Hurt: Secret Diaries of a Junior Doctor, Adam Kay, Picador

Trust Me, I'm a (Junior) Doctor, Max Pemberton, Hodder

Where Does it Hurt? What the Junior Doctor Did Next, Max Pemberton, Hodder

Your Life in My Hands: A Junior Doctor's Story, Rachel Clarke, Metro Publishing

Genetics

The Blind Watchmaker, Richard Dawkins, Penguin

The Epigenetics Revolution: How Modern Biology is Rewriting Our Understanding of Genetics, Disease and Inheritance, Nessa Carey, Icon Books

The Gene: An Intimate History, Siddhartha Mukherjee, Vintage

Genome, Matt Ridley, Fourth Estate

Hacking the Code of Life: How Gene Editing will Rewrite Our Futures, Nessa Carey, Icon Books

The Immortal Life of Henrietta Lacks, Rebecca Skloot, Pan Macmillan

The Language of the Genes, Steve Jones, Flamingo

Who's Afraid of Human Cloning? Gregory E. Pence, Rowman and Littlefield

Y: The Descent of Man, Steve Jones, Abacus

Higher education entry

Getting into Oxford & Cambridge, Trotman Education

HEAP 2025: University Degree Course Offers, Trotman Education

How to Complete Your UCAS Application, Trotman Education

Medical science: general

Asimov's New Guide to Science, Isaac Asimov, Penguin

Aspirin: The Extraordinary Story of a Wonder Drug, Diarmuid Jeffreys, Bloomsbury

Don't Die Young, Dr Alice Roberts, Bloomsbury

Everything You Need to Know About Bird Flu and What You Can Do to Prepare For It, Jo Revill, Rodale

The Greatest Benefit to Mankind: A Medical History of Humanity, Roy Porter, Fontana

The Human Brain: A Guided Tour, Susan Greenfield, Phoenix

Human Instinct, Robert Winston, Bantam

The Noonday Demon: An Anatomy of Depression, Andrew Solomon, Vintage

Pain: The Science of Suffering (Maps of the Mind), Patrick Wall, Weidenfeld and Nicolson

Penicillin Man: Alexander Fleming and the Antibiotic Revolution, Kevin Brown, History Press

From Poison Arrows to Prozac: How Deadly Toxins Changed Our Lives Forever, Stanley Feldman, John Blake Publishing

A Short History of Nearly Everything, Bill Bryson, Black Swan

A User's Guide to the Brain, John Ratey, Abacus

The Vaccine Race: How Scientists Used Human Cells to Combat Killer Viruses, Meredith Wadman, Black Swan

Medical ethics

The Body Hunters: Testing New Drugs on the World's Poorest Patients, Sonia Shah, The New Press

Causing Death and Saving Lives: The Moral Problems of Abortion, Infanticide, Suicide, Euthanasia, Capital Punishment, War and Other Life-or-death Choices, Jonathan Glover, Penguin

Medical Ethics: A Very Short Introduction, Tony Hope, OUP

Medical practice

NHS Plc: The Privatisation of Our Health Care, Allyson M. Pollock, Verso

The NHS at 70, Ellen Welch, Pen and Sword History

Websites

All the medical schools have their own websites (see below) and there are numerous useful and interesting medical sites. These can be found using search engines. Particularly informative sites include the following.

- British Medical Association: www.bma.org.uk
- Department of Health & Social Care: www.gov.uk/government/organisations/department-of-health-and-social-care
- General Medical Council: www.gmc-uk.org
- Student BMJ: www.bmj.com/student
- UCAT: www.ucat.ac.uk
- World Health Organization: www.who.int

Financial advice

For information on the financial side of five to six years at medical school, see the student finance pages at www.gov.uk/student-finance. The Health Careers website (www.healthcareers.nhs.uk/career-planning/study-and-training/considering-or-university/financial-support-university) is also a useful gateway resource.

Contact details

Studying in the UK

Aberdeen
School of Medicine, Medical Sciences and Nutrition
University of Aberdeen
Polwarth Building
Foresterhill
Aberdeen AB25 2ZD
Tel: 01224 437923
Email: medadm@abdn.ac.uk
www.abdn.ac.uk/study/undergraduate/degree-programmes/796/A100/medicine-5-years

Anglia Ruskin
Faculty of Medical Science
Chelmsford campus
Michael Salmon Building
Bishop Hall Lane
Chelmsford
Essex CM1 1SQ
Tel: 01245 4931319
www.anglia.ac.uk/study/undergraduate/medicine

Aston
Aston University
Birmingham B4 7ET
Tel: 0121 204 3000
Email: medicalschool@aston.ac.uk
www2.aston.ac.uk/aston-medical-school

Birmingham
College of Medical and Dental Sciences
University of Birmingham
Edgbaston
Birmingham B15 2TT
Tel: 0121 414 3344
Email: mdsenquiries@contacts.bham.ac.uk
www.birmingham.ac.uk/university/colleges/mds/index.aspx

Brighton and Sussex Medical School
BSMS Teaching Building
University of Sussex
Brighton BN1 9PX
Tel: 01273 606755
Email: information@sussex.ac.uk
www.bsms.ac.uk

Bristol Medical School
University of Bristol
69 St Michael's Hill
Bristol BS2 8DZ
Tel: 0117 331 1831
Email: choosebristol-ug@bristol.ac.uk
www.bris.ac.uk/medical-school

Buckingham Medical School
The University of Buckingham
Hunter Street
Buckingham MK18 1EG
Tel: 01280 814080
Email: medicine-admissions@buckingham.ac.uk
https://medvle.buckingham.ac.uk

Cambridge
University of Cambridge School of Clinical Medicine
Box 111 Cambridge Biomedical Campus
Cambridge CB2 0SP
Tel: 01223 336700
Email: admissions@cam.ac.uk
www.medschl.cam.ac.uk

Cardiff
School of Medicine
UHW Main Building
Heath Park
Cardiff CF14 4XN
Tel: 029 2087 4000
Email: medicine@cardiff.ac.uk
www.cardiff.ac.uk/medicine

Dundee
University of Dundee
Ninewells Hospital
Dundee DD1 9SY
Tel: 01382 383617
Email: asrs-medicine@dundee.ac.uk
www.dundee.ac.uk/undergraduate/medicinek

East Anglia
Norwich Medical School
Faculty of Medicine and Health Sciences
University of East Anglia
Norwich NR4 7TJ
Tel: 01603 591515
Email: enquiries@uea.ac.uk
www.uea.ac.uk/med

Edge Hill
Edge Hill University
St Helen's Road
Ormskirk L39 4QP
Tel: 01695 575171
Email: admissions@edgehill.ac.uk
www.edgehill.ac.uk/study/undergraduate/medicine

Edinburgh
University of Edinburgh
The Queen's Medical Research Institute
47 Little France Crescent
Edinburgh EH16 4TJ
Tel: 0131 242 9100
Email: medug@ed.ac.uk
www.ed.ac.uk/medicine-vet-medicine/edinburgh-medical-school

Exeter
University of Exeter Medical School
St Luke's Campus
Heavitree Road
Exeter EX1 2LU
Tel: 01392 725500
Email: HLS-SROps@exeter.ac.uk
http://medicine.exeter.ac.uk

Glasgow
College of Medical, Veterinary and Life Sciences
Wolfson Medical School Building
University of Glasgow
University Avenue
Glasgow G12 8QQ
Tel: 0141 330 6216
Email: med-sch-admissions@glasgow.ac.uk
www.gla.ac.uk/colleges/mvls

Hull York
Hull York Medical School
Allam Medical Buildings
University of Hull
Hull HU6 7RX
or
Hull York Medical School
John Hughlings Jackson Building
University of York
Heslington
York YO10 5DD
Tel: 0870 124 5500
Email: admissions@hyms.ac.uk
www.hyms.ac.uk

Imperial College London
Faculty of Medicine
Imperial College London
Level 2, Faculty Building
South Kensington Campus
London SW7 2AZ
Tel: 020 7594 7259
Email: medicine.ug.admissions@imperial.ac.uk
www.ic.ac.uk/medicine

Keele
School of Medicine
David Weatherall Building
Keele University
Staffordshire ST5 5BG
Tel: 01782 733937
Email: medicine@keele.ac.uk
www.keele.ac.uk/medicine

King's College London
King's College London
Strand
London WC2R 2LS
Tel: 020 7836 5454
www.kcl.ac.uk/medicine

Kent and Medway
Kent and Medway Medical School
Augustine House
Canterbury CT2 7NZ
Tel: 01227 768896
email: futuredoctors@kmms.ac.uk
https://kmms.ac.uk

Lancaster
Lancaster Medical School
Lancaster University
Lancaster LA1 4YW
Tel: 01524 594595
Email: medicine@lancaster.ac.uk
www.lancaster.ac.uk/lms

Leeds
University of Leeds
Worsley Building
Leeds LS2 9NL
Tel: 0113 343 2336
Email: ugmadmissions@leeds.ac.uk
https://medicinehealth.leeds.ac.uk

Leicester
University of Leicester Medical School
George Davies Centre
Lancaster Road
Leicester LE1 7HA
Tel: 0116 252 2969/2985/3015
Email: med-admis@le.ac.uk
www2.le.ac.uk/departments/msce/undergraduate/medicine

Lincoln
University of Lincoln
Brayford Pool
Lincoln LN6 7TS
Tel: 01522 882000
www.lincoln.ac.uk/home/course/mdcmdcub

Liverpool
School of Medicine
MBChB Office
Cedar House
Ashton Street
Liverpool L69 3GE
Tel: 0151 795 4362
Email: mbchb@liverpool.ac.uk
www.liverpool.ac.uk/medicine

Manchester
Faculty of Biology, Medicine and Health
University of Manchester
Oxford Road
Manchester M13 9PL
Tel: 0161 306 0211
Email: ug.medicine@manchester.ac.uk
www.medicine.manchester.ac.uk

Newcastle
School of Medical Education
Newcastle University
Newcastle upon Tyne NE1 7RU
Tel: 0191 208 6000
Email: medic.ugadmin@ncl.ac.uk
www.ncl.ac.uk/sme/study/undergraduate

Nottingham
Faculty of Medicine and Health Sciences
University of Nottingham
Queen's Medical Centre
Nottingham NG7 2HA
Tel: 0115 823 0141
www.nottingham.ac.uk/mhs

Oxford
Medical Sciences Divisional Office
University of Oxford
John Radcliffe Hospital
Headley Way
Oxford OX3 9DU
Tel: 01865 285790
Email: communications@medsci.ox.ac.uk
www.medsci.ox.ac.uk

Plymouth
Faculty of Medicine and Dentistry
John Bull Building
Plymouth Science Park
Research Way
Plymouth PL6 8BU
Tel: 01752 600600
Email: meddent-admissions@plymouth.ac.uk
www.plymouth.ac.uk/schools/peninsula-medical-school

Queen's Belfast
School of Medicine, Dentistry and Biomedical Sciences
Whitla Medical Building
97 Lisburn Road
Belfast BT9 7BL
Tel: 028 9097 2215
www.qub.ac.uk/schools/mdbs

Queen Mary (Barts and The London School of Medicine and Dentistry)
Garrod Building 4
Newark Street
Whitechapel
London E1 2AT
Tel: 020 7882 5555
Email: smdadmissions@qmul.ac.uk
www.smd.qmul.ac.uk

St Andrews
School of Medicine
University of St Andrews
North Haugh
St Andrews KY16 9TF
Tel: 01334 463599
Email: medicine@st-andrews.ac.uk
https://medicine.st-andrews.ac.uk

St George's
St George's, University of London
Cranmer Terrace
London SW17 0RE
Tel: 020 8672 9944
www.sgul.ac.uk

Sheffield
The Medical School
University of Sheffield
Beech Hill Road
Sheffield S10 2RX
Tel: 0114 222 5522
Email: med-school@sheffield.ac.uk
www.shef.ac.uk/medicine

Southampton
Faculty of Medicine
University of Southampton
12 University Road
Southampton SO17 1BJ
Tel: 023 8059 5571
Email: ugapply.fm@southampton.ac.uk
www.southampton.ac.uk/medicine

Sunderland
The University of Sunderland
Edinburgh Building
City Campus Chester Road
Sunderland SR1 3SD
Tel: 0191 515 2000
Email: student.helpline@sunderland.ac.uk
www.sunderland.ac.uk/about/school-of-medicine

Swansea
Swansea University Medical School
Grove Building
Institute of Life Science
Swansea SA2 8QA
Tel: 01792 602697
Email: studt@swansea.ac.uk
www.swan.ac.uk/medicine

Three Counties
(St John's Campus)
University of Worcester
Henwick Grove
Worcester WR2 6AJ
Tel: 01905 855000
Email: communications@worc.ac.uk
www.worcester.ac.uk/about/academic-schools/medical-school

University College London
UCL Medical School
74 Huntley Street
London WC1E 6BT
Tel: 020 3108 8235/7674/6185
Email: medicaladmissions@ucl.ac.uk
www.ucl.ac.uk/medicalschool

UCLAN
University of Central Lancashire
Fylde Road
Preston PR1 2HE
Tel: 01772 210210
Email: cenquiries@uclan.ac.uk
www.uclan.ac.uk/courses/bachelor_medicine_bachelor_surgery.php

Warwick
Warwick Medical School
University of Warwick
Coventry CV4 7HL
Tel: 02476 574880
Email: wmsinfo@warwick.ac.uk
www2.warwick.ac.uk/fac/med

Volunteering

British Red Cross
44 Moorfields
London EC2Y 9AL
Tel: 0344 871 1111
Email: contactus@redcross.org.uk
www.redcross.org.uk/Get-involved/Volunteer

Do-it (database for volunteering placements)
www.do-it.org.uk

NHS Volunteering
www.england.nhs.uk/participation/get-involved/volunteering

Positive East (HIV/AIDS volunteering)
159 Mile End Road
London E1 4AQ
Tel: 020 7791 2855
Email: talktome@positiveeast.org.uk
www.positiveeast.org.uk

vInspired
Unit 3, 9 Albert Embankment
London SE1 7SP
Tel: 020 7960 7000
Email: info@vinspired.com
https://vinspired.com

Volunteering Matters
The Levy Centre
18–24 Lower Clapton Road
London E5 0PD
Tel: 020 3780 5870
https://volunteeringmatters.org.uk

It is worthwhile contacting your local county or borough council and local hospital to find out what volunteering opportunities it has, for example, in hospitals, care homes or schools (all of which will require criminal record DBS checks).

Health careers

www.healthcareers.nhs.uk/career-planning/career-planning/getting-experience/getting-experience

Working abroad

www.workingabroad.com/project-finder
www.globalpremeds.com/gap-medics

Tables

Table 8 Medical school admissions policies for 2024–25

Institution	Usual offer	Required A level subjects	Retakes considered	Minimum GCSE requirements
Aberdeen	AAA (IB 36 points with 3 at HL, Grade 6)	Chemistry plus one from Biology, Maths and Physics	Only with extenuating circumstances	6/B in English Language and Maths required. Combination of grades 9–6 (A*–B) are expected
Anglia Ruskin	AAA (IB 36 points, 6,6,6 at HL Biology and/or Chemistry, plus one other science)	Chemistry or Biology and one of Biology, Chemistry, Maths or Physics	Yes, resit grades of AAA will be accepted if taken within two academic years prior to the time of application	Five at grade 9–6 (A*–B), including English Language, Maths and 2 sciences
Aston	AAA (IB 37 points, with 7,6,6 at HL including 7 in Chemistry or Biology)	Biology and Chemistry	Yes, but only one resit attempt considered; reasons for resitting must be outlined in the UCAS reference	Minimum of six at 6/B or above. Must include English Language, Maths, Chemistry, Biology or Double Science
Birmingham	A*AA (IB min. 32 points, with HL 7,6,6 including Biology, Chemistry and one other)	Biology and Chemistry	Only with extenuating circumstances	At least seven, including English Language, Maths, Biology and Chemistry, at 6/B
Brighton and Sussex	AAA (IB 36 points, with 6, 6 in Biology and Chemistry)	Biology and Chemistry	Yes, if narrowly missed by one grade in one subject	6/B or above in Maths and English Language or Literature
Bristol	AAA (IB 36 points with 18 points at HL including 6s in Chemistry and one of Biology, Physics or Maths)	Chemistry and either Biology, Physics, Maths or Further Maths	Yes	7/A in Maths, 4/C in English Language
Brunel (non-UK students only)	AAB (IB 36 points, 6,5 in Chemistry or Biology, plus 5 in Chemistry, Biology, Physics or Maths)	Chemistry or Biology plus one from Chemistry, Biology, Physics or Maths	Considered on a case-by-case basis where there have been genuine extenuating circumstances	At least 5/B in Maths and at least 4/C in English Language
Buckingham	ABB (IB 34 points, with 6,6 in Biology and Chemistry)	Chemistry or Biology	Yes, if BBB at first attempt	None
Cambridge	A*A*A (IB 40–42 with HL 7,7,6)	Chemistry and one from Biology, Physics or Maths, although 3 sciences/maths are preferred	In extenuating circumstances	None

Note: *Details were correct when going to press – check websites for updated information.*

Table 8 Continued

Institution	Usual offer	Required A level subjects	Retakes considered	Minimum GCSE requirements
Cardiff	AAA (IB 36 points, including 7,6,6, with 6,6 in HL Biology and Chemistry)	Biology and Chemistry	Only with extenuating circumstances	Must have 6/B in Biology, Chemistry, English Language and Maths
Central Lancashire (UCLAN)	AAA	At least two science subjects, including Chemistry	No	No specific requirements, but evidence of broad study of science, English and Maths
Dundee	AAA (IB 37 points, with 6,6,6 at HL, including HL Chemistry and another science)	Chemistry and one other science	No	Biology, Maths and English at 6/B if not studied at A level
East Anglia	AAA (IB 36 points, with 6,6,6 in all HL subjects, including Biology or Chemistry)	Biology or Chemistry	Yes (ABB or AAC or equivalent from first sitting); an A* will form part of the offer	Six at 7/A or above to include Maths and two sciences, with English Language at 6/B
Edge Hill	AAA (IB 36 points, with 6 in Biology and Chemistry and one other subject)	Biology and Chemistry	Yes	At least five at 6/B to include Biology, Chemistry, English Language and Maths
Edinburgh	A*AA (IB 40 points, with HL 6,6,7 including Chemistry and one other science)	Chemistry (A*) and one of Biology, Maths or Physics	No, unless under there are extenuating circumstances	7/A in Biology, Chemistry, English, Maths
Exeter	AAA (IB 36 points, with 6,6,6 overall to include Biology and Chemistry at HL)	Chemistry and Biology	Yes	4/C in English Language
Glasgow	AAA (IB 38 points, with 6 in HL Biology and Chemistry)	Chemistry and one of Biology, Maths or Physics	Only with extenuating circumstances	English Language at 6/B or above
Hull York	AAB (IB 36 points,with 6,6,5 at HL, including Biology and Chemistry)	Biology and Chemistry	Yes, if achieved BBB at first sitting and taken in one extra year	Six at 9/A* to 4/C; English Language and Maths at 6/B
Imperial	A*AA–AAA (IB 38 points, with 6 in HL Biology and Chemistry)	Chemistry and Biology	Only if the candidate has applied for mitigating circumstances	6/B in English Language
Keele	A*AA (IB 37 points, with 7/6 in all HL subjects, including Biol-ogy or Chemistry and another science)	Biology or Chemistry and another science (including Psychology) or Economics or Maths	Only if applying after total of three years of A level study with achieved grades	Five at 7/A, with Maths, English Language and Science at 6/B or above

Note: *Details were correct when going to press – check websites for updated information.*

Table 8 Continued

Institution	Usual offer	Required A level subjects	Retakes considered	Minimum GCSE requirements
Kent and Medway	AAB (IB 34 points, with 6 in Biology and/or Chemistry and another science)	Chemistry and/or Biology, plus one of Chemistry, Biology, Maths, Physics, Psychology or Computer Science	Only with extenuating circumstances	At least five at 9–6/A*–B, including English Language, Maths, Biology, Chemistry and Physics
King's	A*AA (IB 35 points, with 7,6,6 at HL in Biology and Chemistry)	Biology and Chemistry	Only with extenuating circumstances	B/6 in English Language and Maths
Lancaster	AAA (IB 36 points, with HL 6,6,6 including 6 in any two of Biology, Chemistry and Psychology)	Two of Biology, Chemistry and Psychology	Yes, if achieved ABB at first attempt	Eight, including 6/B in Biology, Chemistry, Physics, English Language and Maths. All others at 4/C or above
Leeds	AAA (IB 36 points, three HL grade 6, one from Biology or Chemistry)	Chemistry or Biology (if no Chemistry, Physics or Maths must be taken)	Only with extenuating circumstances	Six at minimum grade 6/B, including Chemistry and Biology, English Language and Maths
Leicester	AAA (IB 34 points, with 7,6,6 in three HL subjects, including Chemistry or Biology plus one from Biology, Chemistry, Maths, Physics or Psychology)	Chemistry or Biology, and one from Biology, Chemistry, Maths, Physics or Psychology	Only with extenuating circumstances	6/B in English Language, Maths and two sciences
Lincoln	AAA (IB 36 points, with 6 in all HL subjects including Biology and Chemistry)	Biology and Chemistry	Yes, if ABB at first sitting with A in Biology or Chemistry	Six at 7/A including Biology and Chemistry, with 6/B in Maths and English Language
Liverpool	AAA (IB 36 points, with 6,6,6 in HL Chemistry with either Biology, Physics or Maths)	Chemistry, with either Biology, Physics or Mathematics	Yes, with ABB at first sitting	Nine, including Biology, Chemistry, Physics, English Language and Maths. Score must be better than 15 for best nine subjects, with 7/8/9/A*/A = 2 and 6/B = 1
Manchester	AAA (IB 36 points with at least 6,6,6 at HL with Chemistry or Biology plus another science)	Chemistry or Biology and one from Chemistry, Biology, Physics, Psychology, Maths or Further Maths	Yes, if ABB at first attempt, with A*A*A expected after resit	Seven GCSEs at A/7 or above. Including English Language, Maths and 2 sciences at minimum 6/B
Newcastle	AAA (IB 36 points with at least 5 in all subjects)	None	One subject can be repeated once. An A* will be expected	None

***Note:** Details were correct when going to press – check websites for updated information.*

Table 8 Continued

Institution	Usual offer	Required A level subjects	Retakes considered	Minimum GCSE requirements
Nottingham	AAA (IB 36 points, with 6 in HL subjects inc. Biology and Chemistry)	Biology and Chemistry	Yes, but for no more than two A levels if ABB at first attempt, with A in Biology or Chemistry	Six at 7/A, As to include Chemistry, Biology and English Language and Maths at 6/B
Oxford	A*AA (IB 39 points, with HL 7,6,6, including Chemistry and one other science)	Chemistry and one from Biology, Physics or Maths	Potentially, but contact university for specific advice	No specific requirements
Plymouth	A*AA–AAA (IB 36–38 points, with 6 in HL Biology plus one other science from Chemistry, Maths, Physics and Psychology)	Biology and one from Chemistry, Physics, Maths and Psychology	Yes if ABB at first attempt, otherwise can apply as resit with achieved grades	Seven at 9–4/A*–C, including English Language, Maths and two sciences
Queen Mary, University of London	A*AA (IB 38 points with 6,6,6 in HL subjects including Biology or Chemistry and a second science or Maths)	Biology or Chemistry plus a second science from Chemistry, Biology, Physics and Maths	Only with extenuating circumstances	English Language, Biology, Chemistry and Maths included in profile of 7,7,7,6,6,6 or A,A,A,B,B,B
Queen's Belfast	A*AA/AAA (IB 36 points, with 6,6,6 in HL subjects to include Biology and Chemistry)	Chemistry and Biology	If previously accepted Queen's offer and missed by one grade (A*AB)	Scored on best nine subjects, so high grades will be advantageous. Maths and Physics at 4/C if not offered at AS or A level
St Andrews	AAA (IB 38 points with HL 6,6,6)	Chemistry and one from Biology, Physics or Maths	With extenuating circumstances if close to meeting entry requirements	Five at 7/A
St George's	A*AA–AAA (IB 36 points with 18 points at HL and 6 in Biology and Chemistry)	Biology and Chemistry	No	Five at 6/B or above, including English Language, Maths and Science
Sheffield	AAA (IB 36 points with 6 in HL subjects including Chemistry or Biology or one other science subject)	Chemistry or Biology and one other from Chemistry, Biology, Physics, Psychology or Maths	Yes	At least five at 7/A, including at least 6/B in Maths, English Language and the sciences
Southampton	AAA (IB 36 points, with 6 in HL subjects including Biology and one other science)	Biology and one other science	Yes	Seven at 6/B, including Maths, Biology Chemistry and English Language
Sunderland	AAA (IB points 35, 6,6,6 in HL subjects to include Chemistry or Biology and one other science)	Biology or Chemistry and a second science	Yes if ABB at first attempt	Five at 7/A with 6/B in English language, Maths, Biology, Chemistry and Physics
UCL	A*AA (IB 39, with 19 in HL subjects, including Biology and Chemistry)	Biology and Chemistry	No	6/B in English Language and Maths

Note: *Details were correct when going to press – check websites for updated information.*

Table 9 Medical school interview and written test policies for 2024–25

Institution	Type and typical length (minutes)	Pre-admissions test	Information on how UCAT is used
Aberdeen	MMI	UCAT	UCAT cut-off score is not used. No strict ranking of scores. In 2022–23, lowest UK score interviewed was 2500.
Anglia Ruskin	MMI	UCAT	Applicants are ranked according to score. SJT band 4 will be rejected.
Aston	MMI	UCAT	Considered alongside the other entry requirements. No cut-off score.
Birmingham	MMI	UCAT	No minimum cut-off, but performance will be given a score that will contribute to the overall application score. SJT band will be used at the interview stage.
Brighton and Sussex	MMI	To be decided	n/a
Bristol	MMI	UCAT	Combined score used to select interviewees. For 2023 entry the threshold was 2910, but this changes each year.
Brunel (international students only)	MMI	UCAT/ GAMSAT	No UCAT cut-off score, but SJT band 4 is rejected.
Buckingham	MMI	None	n/a
Cambridge	Panel, 2 interviews each 25-30 minutes	To be decided	n/a
Cardiff	MMI	UCAT/ GAMSAT	Used holistically as part of the selection process, but no strict cut-off.
Chester (graduate-entry only)	MMI	UCAT/ GAMSAT	Threshold varies from year to year. For 2024 entry, UCAT threshold was 2540
Dundee	MMI	UCAT	No minimum cut-off score.
East Anglia	MMI	UCAT	No cut-off score, but a high score is advantageous.
Edge Hill	MMI	UCAT	Scores are ranked, and there is a cut off to select for interview. SJT band 4 is immediately rejected.
Edinburgh	Assessment day, including MMI	UCAT	UCAT scores are ranked; in 2024, cut off was 2470. SJT band 4 will not be considered.
Exeter	MMI	UCAT/ GAMSAT	UCAT score receives 25% weighting. Academic achievement receives the other 75%.

Table 9 Continued

Institution	Type and typical length (minutes)	Pre-admissions test	Information on how UCAT is used
Glasgow	Panel, 2 interviews over 30 minutes	UCAT	Interviews are allocated accordingly by UCAT score for those that meet all other criteria.
Hull-York	MMI	UCAT	Total score plus SJT band is given a points score to be used alongside GCSE results and contextual data. SJT band 4 is not accepted.
Imperial	MMI	To be decided	n/a
Keele	MMI	UCAT	A total score below 2280 or SJT band 4 will not be considered.
Kent Medway	MMI	UCAT	There is a minimum threshold for total UCAT score, although it is described as 'generous'.
King's	MMI	UCAT	The overall average score and SJT are taken into account when shortlisting candidates, but there is no cut-off score.
Lancaster	MMI	To be decided	n/a
Leeds	MMI	UCAT	Information not yet aavailable.
Leicester	MMI	UCAT	Total score is used in combination with academic attainment to rank for interview. SJT band 4 is not accepted.
Lincoln	MMI	UCAT	No fixed UCAT threshold. SJT band 4 is not accepted.
Liverpool	MMI	UCAT/ GAMSAT	No fixed threshold, but performance is used as an indicator for inviting to interview.
Manchester	MMI	UCAT	Threshold for interview varies each year according to national performance; in 2022–23 the threshold was 2750.
Newcastle	MMI (Home) Panel (International)	UCAT	Students above threshold score who meet academic requirements are invited to interview. 2022 threshold was 2870.
Nottingham	MMI	UCAT	UCAT score is used for interview selection. There is no fixed threshold. SJT band 4 is not accepted.
Oxford	Panel (interviews at two colleges)	To be decided	n/a
Plymouth	MMI	UCAT/ GAMSAT	Score must be above threshold. For 2023 entry, this was 2680.

Table 9 Continued

Institution	Type and typical length (minutes)	Pre-admissions test	Information on how UCAT is used
Queen Mary	Panel	UCAT	Score weighted with academic profile. In 2022–23 the cut-off score was 2720.
Queen's Belfast	MMI	UCAT	Score used alongside GCSE profile to rank for interview.
ScotGEM (Graduate only)	MMI	GAMSAT	n/a
Sheffield	MMI	UCAT	Scores below 2440 are rejected. All other scores are ranked to determine who is invited to interview.
Southampton	Selection day, interview and group task	UCAT	Scores ranked to determine who is invited to interview.
St Andrews	MMI	UCAT	If application has met academic criteria, UCAT score is then ranked, with approximately top 500 invited to interview.
St George's	MMI	UCAT	Thresholds for overall score must be met; in 2022–23 the threshold was 2630.
Sunderland	MMI and a maths test	UCAT	UCAT score must be within top 8 deciles of the cohort, with SJT band 1–3.
Surrey (graduate-entry only)	MMI	UCAT/ GAMSAT	Scores are ranked to determine who is interviewed.
Swansea (graduate-entry only)	Panel (2 interviews with 30-minute written test)	GAMSAT	n/a
UCL	MMI	To be decided	n/a
UCLAN	MMI	UCAT (Home students only)	UCAT score used as part of the selection process.
Ulster (graduate-entry only)	MMI	GAMSAT	n/a
Warwick (graduate-entry only)	MMI	UCAT	Total score required for interview varies from year to year. Need to achieve at least the overall mean on the VR subtest.
Worcester (graduate-entry only)	Panel (2 interviews)	UCAT/ GAMSAT	UCAT must be passed to a requisite level. No further details are provided.

Source: UCAS website, University websites and Medical Schools Council website; correct at time of going to print.

Glossary

AIDS (acquired immune deficiency syndrome)
AIDS is a disease that affects the immune system, lowering the body's resistance to infection. The disease is caused by the human immunodeficiency virus (HIV).

BHA (British Humanist Association)
The association acting for those who are non-religious who seek to live ethical lives on the basis of reason and humanity.

BMA (British Medical Association)
The professional medical association and trade union for doctors and medical students.

BMI (body mass index)
Indicates whether someone is overweight or underweight, based on their weight and height.

CBL (Case-based learning)
The medical training that some medical schools use that is more case led, based on clinical examples, than the more problem-based learning courses.

CSP (Chartered Society of Physiotherapists)
Professional, educational and trade union body for the UK's physiotherapy workforce.

GAMSAT (Graduate Medical School Admissions Test)
A test introduced in 1999 by some universities to aid in the selection of candidates who already have degrees.

GEP (Graduate Entry Programme)
A four-year programme offered by universities for students who already have a degree, as opposed to the traditional five-year programme.

GMC (General Medical Council)
The governing body that protects, promotes and maintains the health and safety of the public by ensuring proper standards in the practice of medicine.

Integrated courses
Those where basic medical sciences are taught concurrently with clinical studies. Thus, this style is a compromise between a traditional course and a PBL course.

Intercalated degree
An intercalated degree is a one-year course of study after the pre-clinical years to attain a further degree, e.g. in biochemistry or anatomy.

MB (Bachelor of Medicine)
One of the three degrees that can be awarded by medical schools to students after four or five years of academic study.

MBBS (Bachelor of Medicine and Surgery)
One of the three degrees that can be awarded by medical schools to students after four or five years of academic study.

MBChB
Some medical schools award this degree instead of the MBBS. This depends on the medical school.

MMR (measles, mumps and rubella)
A vaccination given to young children around the age of one.

MRI (magnetic resonance imaging)
A medical imaging technique used in radiology to visualise detailed internal structures of the body.

MRSA (methicillin-resistant *Staphylococcus aureus*)
A bacterium responsible for several difficult-to-treat infections in humans. It is also called multidrug-resistant bacteria.

NICE (National Institute for Health and Care Excellence)
NICE sets standards for quality healthcare and produces guidance on medicines, treatments and procedures.

PBL (problem-based learning)
The medical training that some medical schools use and is a more patient-oriented approach than the more traditional lecture styles.

Personal statement
The written document provided by the candidate about themselves, which is part of the UCAS application.

PLAB
The Professional Linguistic and Assessments Board sets a test for assessing eligibility for students entering the UK to practise medicine having studied abroad.

Student BMJ
A publication produced for medical students.

UCAS (Universities and Colleges Admissions Service)
The central body through which students apply to medical school or any higher education institution.

UCAS codes
The identifying letters and numbers of the various university courses. These are vital when making your application. Medical courses range from A100 to A104 depending on previous experience (e.g. A levels, degree, etc.).

UCAT (University Clinical Aptitude Test)
An application test that certain medical schools require students to sit before accepting them onto the course. See Table 4 on page 55 for a list of which universities require this test.

WHO (World Health Organization)
A specialised agency of the United Nations that acts as a coordinating authority on international public health.

Work experience
Voluntary work (normally) organised before you apply to medical school which is described in your personal statement. This is a vital component of your application.